Patient Listening

Patient Listening

A Doctor's Guide

Edited by Loreen Herwaldt

University of Iowa Press, Iowa City

University of Iowa Press, Iowa City 52242

Copyright © 2008 by the University of Iowa Press

www.uiowapress.org

Printed in the United States of America

Design by April Leidig-Higgins

The University of Iowa Press is a member of Green Press Initiative and is committed to preserving natural resources.

Printed on acid-free paper

LCCN: 2007940202

ISBN-13: 978-1-58729-652-9

ISBN-10: 1-58729-652-7

08 09 10 11 12 P 5 4 3 2 1

Patient Listening is dedicated to the authors
who shared their stories with me. In particular,
this work is dedicated to the memories of
Laura Evans, who died on October 17, 2000,
of a glioblastoma; Michael Gearin-Tosh, who
died July 29, 2005; Sekou Sundiata, who died
July 18, 2007; and to Christina Middlebrook,
who was very ill when this book went to press.

The patient must be interviewed. By means of these questions it is just possible to learn a great deal concerning illness, which enables a better treatment. The time that the illness began is also important. In addition, one should inquire as to the patient's attitude toward life and general mental state. In this way, the patient's health can be assessed.

— Rufus of Ephesus, first century A.D.

Lorrie, Lorrie, there's a person under there, there's a person under there!

— Catherine Powell Herwaldt, summer 1969

Contents

Acknowledgments

When we were first married, my husband would sing several lines from David Bryne's song "Once in a Lifetime": "And you may find yourself in a beautiful house, with a beautiful wife / And you may ask yourself—Well... How did I get here?" Both of us were surprised to find ourselves married to each other. I am similarly surprised to be publishing a book of found poems. *Patient Listening* is both a product of relationships and about relationships, and I could not have created this book without help from many people. I would like to acknowledge those who helped me craft this surprise.

Mary Swander started me on this journey with her memoir *Out of This World: A Woman's Life among the Amish*, helped me find *St. Benedict's Rule for Monasteries* and St. John's Abbey, and suggested that I create a performance piece from my found poems using Anna Deavere Smith's *Fires in the Mirror* as a model.

A Whole New Life: An Illness and a Healing by Reynolds Price pushed me to seek additional narratives of illness and to dream about a sabbatical project that would allow me to meet the authors.

Todd Wiblin and Karen Kuntz invited me to a Sunday school class on lectio divina, which reminded me of Kathleen Norris's book *The Cloister Walk*, which in turn led me to the Institute for Ecumenical and Cultural Research at St. John's Abbey.

The Institute and St. John's University and Monastery provided a beautiful environment and a prayerful daily structure that encouraged me to read, to reflect, and to listen. Patrick Henry, Father Kilian McDonald, my fellow resident scholars in the class of 2000, and the audience at my public lecture gave me the impetus I needed to begin creating *Patient Listening* and the opportunity to present a nascent version.

Kristi Ferguson and Marcy Rosenbaum suggested that first-year medical students present *Patient Listening* as readers' theater, made a place for it in a crowded curriculum, and helped me choose the final found poems and create the users' guide. Numerous first-year medical students at the University of Iowa Carver College of Medicine have given life to the piece through their inspired readings.

Richard Caplan, Robert Sherertz, Richard LeBlond, Peter Densen, James Martins, Martin Kohn, and Carol Donley created opportunities to present *Patient Listening* to residents, physicians in private practices, internists at academic medical centers, and health-care workers in different disciplines, all of whom gave me valuable feedback.

Dale Hancock, Barbara Herwaldt, David Herwaldt, Jean Pottinger, Rebecca Porter, Marge Murray, Carol Donley, Kristi Ferguson, Marcy Rosenbaum, and Mary Nilsen critically read part or all of *Patient Listening* and suggested ways to improve it.

Writing teachers Mary Nilsen, Marilyn Abildskov, Nancy Barry, and Marge Murray enabled me to write the introductory essay. Marc Nieson taught me the writing exercise that led me to create the first found poem from a story one of the authors told me.

Susan Felch gave me a name for the genre I stumbled upon while using Marc Nieson's writing exercise.

As my mentors, Suzanne Poirier and Richard Frankel encouraged me, pushed me to go deeper, and introduced me to essential resources.

David Morris and Julie Reichert believed in the project and in me. They encouraged me to continue the project.

The Bayer Institute for Healthcare Communication provided funding and connected me with Richard Frankel.

The University of Iowa allowed me to take a sabbatical to do this project.

Kelly Smith, Stephanie Ryan, and Mary Beckler transcribed hours and hours of interviews.

Twenty-four gifted writers generously shared their time and stories with me and allowed me to shape their stories into found poems and then share the found poems with you.

Holly Carver and Joseph Parsons both thought my idea was really strange but they kept reading and decided it was worth publishing. They patiently answered my questions and helped me shape the final version.

Marc Abbott, my husband, introduced me to Reynolds Price by suggesting I read a published interview, drove thousands of miles so that I could interview the authors, read multiple versions of *Patient Listening*, and gave me the freedom to pursue my dream. He supported and loved me from start to finish.

Patient Listening

Introduction

Have you ever walked into the pocket of a revolving door and come out the other side different than when you entered? Or have you been going about your daily life, minding your own business, when suddenly a white rabbit with pink eyes catches your attention and for some reason you feel deeply, but cannot explain why, you follow him into his hole and, after a long free fall, you land in a new world populated by all sorts of interesting characters who coax you to do or be something you had never even imagined before? I have. In 1994, my life took such an unexpected turn. As I look back on it, the metaphor that best describes the experience is Alice's tumble through the rabbit hole. *Patient Listening* is the fruit of my time in Wonderland.

In June of 1987, I began my first real job as a faculty member at the University of Iowa College of Medicine. Before that, I had made all the right professional moves. I graduated high in my medical school class and then spent twelve years in apprenticeships: three years in a strenuous internal-medicine residency program at Barnes Hospital, two years at the Centers for Disease Control and Prevention investigating outbreaks of gastroenteritis and Pontiac Fever, and five years as a clinical and research fellow in infectious diseases at Washington University. All of these experiences prepared me to be a faculty member at a respected medical school.

I spent the next years at Iowa building an academic career in infectious diseases and hospital epidemiology — not exactly the standard bench research track to the coveted prize of tenure, but close enough. I was treading the path, albeit a circuitous one, to a traditional, safe career in academic medicine: seeing patients; teaching students, residents, and fellows; getting grants; doing research; publishing so I wouldn't perish. But I became restless as I progressed along that path, merely ticking off the milestones. I felt vaguely unsettled, as if what I was doing wasn't really why I went to medical school. I began asking myself Peggy Lee's question, "Is that all there is?"

Then one day in the fall of 1994, I was walking down a flight of stairs at a local bookstore when I saw a display of new releases. A photograph of Amish dresses hanging on a clothesline drew my eye to a book entitled *Out of This World: A Journey of Healing*, by a local writer Mary Swander. The cover photograph intrigued me, and the blurb on the back hooked me with its mention of "a severe allergic illness" that forced the author to move to the Amish area near Iowa City and to grow her own food. I bought the book not knowing at the time that my career and life were about to take an unexpected turn.

I couldn't stop reading *Out of This World*. I wanted to know more about the bad experiences Ms. Swander had while receiving medical care, and I had the unhappy sense that some had occurred at the hospital where I worked. Soon after, I discovered Reynolds Price's book, *A Whole New Life: An Illness and a Healing*, about his treatment for a malignant tumor in his spinal cord. Price also had very troubling encounters with physicians despite being treated in a prestigious academic medical center.

These two stories drove me to search for personal accounts of illness. Over the course of several years I continued to work my day job, do my research, teach, and care for patients. But I grew more restless, sensing that something was missing from my daily work, that I wasn't doing what I went to medical school to do. At night, I filled the bathtub with hot water, sank my tired body into the bubbles and lavender, and immersed myself in more stories of writers who had been beset by illness. I loved the stories, but I was also disturbed by them. It seemed that each author had had experiences with health-care providers who were right out of the videotapes we show in schools of medicine and nursing to demonstrate how not to interact with patients. At times, I became defensive and angry while reading these stories; I was tired of having my profession bashed in print. At other times, I was saddened and humbled to read how clinicians had hurt patients they were "caring for," and I remembered my own failures. As I read, I became more convinced that persons who had received health care for illnesses, injuries, or disabilities could teach me both what it is like to be a patient and how to communicate with and care for the persons coming to me for diagnosis and treatment.

While soaking in that tub and walking to and from work, I fantasized about meeting these authors and talking with them about their experiences. To realize those dreams, I decided I would interview the authors whose stories I had read to learn more about their experiences of illness, injury, or disability, and also of getting health care for these disorders. I designed a research project that would help me hear patients' stories and voices and experience their perspectives — something medical school, residency, and practice as a physician had not taught me. This would be my own private "patient-language-immersion school," a school in which I would be the student and the authors/patients would be my teachers.

I chose to interview people who had written about being ill because I felt authors who had reflected on these experiences might be able to articulate feelings that for most of us remain buried, inchoate, or inexpressible; and I hoped health-care providers who listened to these narratives could learn to perceive similar feelings in their own patients. Were this to occur, communication between patients and health-care providers would improve and both patients and providers would be more satisfied with their interactions.

During the academic year 1999–2000, I took a sabbatical to meet and interview the authors. Before that time, I sent letters and emails or made phone calls to tell the authors about my project and to ask if they would be willing to speak with me. William Styron's agent wrote to decline my request. Numerous authors did not respond to two or three letters requesting interviews. Their absolute silence left me feeling snubbed and disappointed. These rejections were assuaged by the surprise and delight I felt when many authors said "Yes!" because they were pleased that a doctor wanted to listen to their stories.

I began in July 1999 by interviewing Mary Swander at her home, a renovated, one-room school house with panoramic views of Amish farms, and I finished in January 2005 by interviewing poet, musician, and theater artist Sekou Sundiata at a noisy restaurant in Iowa City. In between, I traveled across the U.S., to Canada, and to England to speak with twenty-two other authors. Richard Selzer met me in the Yale University Library where he writes every day and Jane Smiley talked with me by phone. Some authors, such as the stocking-footed Oliver Sacks, spoke with me in their offices; others invited me into their homes. The authors generously shared their time with me. Jane Smiley talked with me for forty-five minutes; Nancy Mairs, who is quadriplegic, conversed with me for five hours over two days. Most of the other authors spent one to three hours talking with me and some treated me to home-cooked meals.

I prepared extensively for the interviews, rereading the authors' published accounts, taking notes, and writing specific questions in addition to the standard list I took with me to each session. I tried to avoid the machine-gun-like interrogation style some doctors use to elicit information quickly and maintain control of an interview. Instead, I used my list of questions as a loose guide to the issues I hoped to address and I responded as fitting the conversation, not simply with the next question on the list. While I was interviewing, I felt alert and flushed with excitement. I left most interviews elated by the stories I had heard and exhausted from concentrating so intently. Strangely, time seemed elastic. The shortest interviews were long enough to cover my essential questions and even the longest interviews seemed too short.

Initially I had planned to do qualitative analysis on both the published texts and the interview transcripts, but the rabbit hole turned in a direction I had not foreseen. One evening while reading transcripts, I remembered a creative writing exercise in which one writes a paragraph, then deletes words from it, and finally arranges the remaining words on the page like a poem. Designed to help writers find the gist of their meaning and distill the most powerful words from their prose, the exercise taught me to condense long passages by keeping the most salient or provocative words and heightening their effect with line breaks usually reserved for poetry. I used these steps to shape a rambling story one writer told me about grieving for her bones after her hips were replaced with bionic parts. I liked the results. I tried the exercise again with a story the same writer told me about her encounter with a plastic surgeon. Several days later, I read these two "poems" at the end of a seminar I gave about my project. I was rewarded and honored with deep silence when I finished reading. This absolute stillness told me that the "poems" had a concentrated emotional power that the unedited stories did not. Encouraged, I continued to craft "poems" from stories other writers told me about their interactions with health-care workers.

But then I encountered a problem. I had no idea what to call this new form. The end product looked like a poem, but it did not use images. It was part quotation and part distillation from an interview transcript, but it was not quite prose any more. I eventually chose the term "found poem" because I shaped each one from someone else's story, from someone else's words. However, choosing a name for the form did not help me decide what to do with the individual pieces. On Mary Swander's recommendation, I watched and read Anna Deavere Smith's performance piece *Fires in the Mirror*, which gave me the idea to arrange the found poems into a written work that could be read silently by a single person or could be read dramatically by one or more people for an audience.

During these months, I also read about the history, philosophy, and discourse of medicine. As I read, I realized that one major problem in clinician-patient communication is that patients tell doctors and nurses very personal stories, but we health-care providers often respond with technical answers — differential diagnoses, tests to be done, therapies to be tried. Patients often feel unheard and dehumanized by these interactions. I also recognized that my plan to do qualitative analysis on the interview transcripts would recapitulate this very problem. By simply analyzing the texts, I would respond technically to the authors' stories and I would mimic what I was criticizing, what I hoped to avoid in my own practice and teaching. Consequently, instead of doing qualitative analysis during my sabbatical, I read the interview transcripts and responded personally to the stories as I created more found poems and arranged them to form a nascent version of *Patient Listening*.

As I shaped and concentrated the spoken prose into found poems and sent the first-person introductions and the poems back to the authors for their comments, I found myself engaged in an extended dialogue with the individual authors who shared their stories and lives with me. I arranged poems from various authors so that the voices and ideas would interact with each other. Subsequently, medical students and other health-care professionals have interpreted the poems while performing them as readers' theater; audiences have evaluated the performance piece and answered reflection questions. I, in turn, considered the authors' and the audiences' comments as I shaped the final content and form of the piece. The process of assembling the found poems into a coherent whole has been like engaging in a rich multiperson conversation.

Patient Listening comprises twenty-four monologues, each one introduced by a first-person description of an author I interviewed, followed by the found poems relating that person's experiences with doctors, or nurses, or the health-care system. These monologues describe doctors who call their patients by the wrong names, doctors who are late to appointments, doctors who are rude and disrespectful to patients, doctors who have bad bedside and telephone manner, and doctors who won't answer questions. Some of the poems laud nurses who do small acts of kindness like hugging patients in isolation, nurses who help patients accomplish their own goals, nurses whose presence and care help patients regain their sanity, and nurses who help patients make informed decisions about treatments. Others describe nurses who assume patients want pain medication because they are addicted to narcotics, nurses who delay bringing the patients' mail, nurses who ask questions but don't listen to the answers, and nurses who don't trust patients to know their own bodies. Numerous found poems tell of doctors who give patients their undivided attention, doctors who ask open-ended questions and listen to the answers, doctors who listen for clues to what ails a patient, and doctors who help patients learn to manage their own care and to recover their lives. Several found poems recount patients' fears that doctors will tell them bad news during routine checkups or during follow-up visits for cancer. Others record patients' efforts to train their physicians, patients' emotions after losing body parts or seeing their own intestines, and patients' perspectives on evidence-based medicine, alternative medicine, and chemotherapy. A few of the poems even describe the perceptions of doctors who became patients.

No matter their major themes, the poems reveal both the commonness of patients' experiences and desires and the uniqueness of each patient. The patients' individuality is particularly apparent when poems from different authors express contradictory views, showing that physicians and other health professionals must listen to patients and tailor their responses to the particular patient's needs and desires, rather than reciting a prepared empathy script for every patient. The found poems also illustrate simple things health-care workers can do to build relationships and aid healing; they show how just one sentence or one word can destroy even the possibility of a therapeutic relationship. Some poems will inspire and encourage the reader; others are likely to elicit anger, despair, denial, or defensiveness.

As a physician myself, I find the negative stories discomfiting; but I have learned that if I listen to them and let them expose my weaknesses, I can improve my own interactions with patients, and thereby improve my practice and increase my satisfaction. I encourage health-care workers to sit with these critical stories, to listen and learn from them. If we avoid or dismiss them, our practice will suffer and our lives will be the poorer. In fact, physicians who communicate poorly with patients are much more likely than physicians who communicate well to be dissatisfied with their careers and to be sued by disgruntled patients. Moreover, we in health care should be ashamed that medical students actually lose their natural skills in listening and empathizing as they advance through our schools of medicine. We must counteract this tendency by intentionally listening to patients' stories so that we can retune our ears and our hearts to hear our patients' voices.

I did not always value patients' stories. I was, in general, not brusque or rude to patients, but I did not know I needed their stories to help me with my work as a physician. I did not understand that I needed to ask patients to share their goals and stories with me. I am embarrassed to admit I once told a patient, "Don't tell me what you think you have. Tell me your symptoms." Since then, the process of reading the published accounts of illness, interviewing the authors, and creating the poems and the performance piece permanently changed me. I discovered that if I listened carefully, and deeply, I could work more efficiently and effectively and also achieve greater satisfaction for both my patients and myself. I now understand that patients' stories provide essential clues to their diagnoses and to the best treatment options, and that the stories connect us as human beings. I learned to inquire directly about a patient's ideas and beliefs about his diagnosis and to ask what goals he has for this particular visit, for his treatment, and for his life. I learned that the patient is, in a sense, always the physician's teacher.

Physician and writer William Carlos Williams nurtured his ability to hear his patients' stories, deeming this skill vital to good doctoring. Writing about the essential nature of the physician's work, Williams said: "The poem springs from the half-spoken words of such patients as the physician sees from day to day. . . . Humbly he presents himself before it and by long practice he strives as best he can to interpret the manner of its speech. In that the secret lies. This, in the end, comes perhaps to be the occupation of the physician after a lifetime of careful listening."

Creating *Patient Listening* allowed me to hear the poems that authors/patients spoke to me as they recounted experiences with doctors and nurses. Reading these monologues may allow physicians and other health-care workers to hear these poems and stories, and, if they reflect on what they have heard, to better appreciate and elicit their own patients' stories. *Patient Listening* speaks also to patients and their family members. And soon enough, all of us will be patients and family members of patients. To paraphrase Louise De-Salvo, *Patient Listening* says to those needing health care, "You have a story to tell about this illness and this story is critically important to your care."

The authors I interviewed gave me their time and the poems that sprang from their words. I, in turn, offer this gift to you so that you can appreciate the people and the narratives that taught me to welcome patients' stories. I hope you too will be engaged and challenged by their stories as presented by *Patient Listening*. I invite you to enter the conversation.

How to Use This Book

This section of the book is primarily for educators, health-care educators, and those teaching classes on health and illness, health communication, death and dying, and other related fields. Before I describe how this book can be used in education, however, I would say that I hope health-care workers and lay people alike will read this book as they would a play, a collection of poems, or a book of personal essays—for their own enjoyment and edification. I encourage health-care professionals to savor the language and the vivid descriptions, to respond both viscerally and rationally to the stories and the emotions, and to reflect on how they as practitioners can improve their relationships with patients. My hope is that lay people and health-care workers who become patients will recognize their own stories in those articulated by the writers of *Patient Listening* and that this collection will honor and validate their experiences.

Patient Listening is not a traditional pedagogical tool and its subject is not objective hard science (the staple of medical education). Instead, this book provides a counterpoint to the usual health-care curriculum, whatever the level. *Patient Listening* is easy to use; it does not require special equipment, expertise, or space. It requires simply that educators set aside a short period of time in the curriculum to let students hear patients' perspectives on their experiences with health care. Perhaps Tom Sleigh's poem "Medical Education" best illustrates why *Patient Listening* is an important addition to health-care education.

Medical training is
    fantastically narrow and intensive.
    It has to be.

It is all about specialization
    and it reduces people to technicians.
Everything is about the numbers on your chart.

I'm not saying doctors need to
    go to liberal arts college.
But I think it would be important humanly
    for medical students, throughout their training,
        to read about
                        the real experience of people
        to get
                        the patient's point of view,
because these stories educate people
    to have professional compassion,
                    which I don't think they otherwise get.

I have heard people describe
    their experiences of anatomy class,
    of working on a stiff.
Everybody is initially horrified
    and that goes away,
if you don't have anything
                    to counterbalance it.

There are doctors
    who write about their experience
    as doctors.
They have built-in cachet.
Some have written very well
    and others you feel
    are on a power trip.

I think it is important for a good physician
    to be exposed to materials
                    that come directly from patients.

My goal here is to let patients speak for themselves so that health-
care workers can learn simple things to do to improve interactions

with them. I hope the voices on the pages will, as Sleigh suggests, help health-care workers know the suffering of their patients. *Patient Listening* can also help patients understand how important their stories are to their own health care. Perhaps this work will encourage patients to identify which elements of their own stories are essential to their treatment and will at the same time challenge them to seek clinicians who listen attentively.

How I Created This Book

The poems within *Patient Listening* are drawn from transcripts of interviews I conducted with twenty-four authors who had written about their experiences of illness, injury, or disability. I identified their stories about getting health care, removed excess words, and arranged the remaining words as poems on the page. In some cases, I removed very few words. I simply listened to the cadence of the story and placed line breaks where they felt right. In other cases, I imagined I was freeing a sculpture from a massive rock as I removed many words from several paragraphs to create spare poetic forms. I call these creations "found poems" because I created them from other people's words.

After reviewing critiques, and based on my own preferences, I chose found poems that address important issues about the clinician-patient relationship and that elicit powerful responses from readers and audiences. I crafted first-person introductions for each author's poems from information or stories that they shared with me in their interviews or that they included in their published accounts. Finally, I arranged the individual authors' monologues so that the pieces would interact with each other. I tried to achieve a balance of voices: men and women; positive and negative; sober and humorous. I began and concluded the book with found poems describing doctors who honor patients' stories and the effect this has on the patients telling those stories. I intentionally included stories about nurses, doctors, and doctors in particular specialties. I chose stories telling what it is like to get care for a variety of illnesses, injuries, and disabilities. I selected stories about communication, or the lack thereof, between health-care workers and patients. About connecting. Disconnecting.

Medical researchers and clinicians are taught that we must maintain a dispassionate distance from our topics or our patients. We must remain objective so that we do not affect the results of our research or become too attached to our patients. To become involved with the subject or to be subjective is to do bad work. Yet, as originally used in philosophy, the term *objective* did not mean to remain distant from the object of study; it meant to know the object, and to do so one cannot remain distant. Similarly, Sir William Osler's famous term *equinimitas* has been misunderstood by generations of physicians to mean that we must remain aloof from the patients we treat. Rather than meaning physicians or other health-care workers must be untouched by their patients' suffering, *equinimitas* means that we must remain calm or centered in the midst of sorrow or chaos so that we can provide good care.

Throughout the process of creating this volume, I tried to be true to the philosophical meaning of *objective* and to Osler's sense of *equinimitas*. I did not try to remove myself from the stories the authors told me. Instead, I immersed myself in them to learn from the patient — not from physicians, nurses, or medical educators — what it is like to get health care. I also interacted extensively with the stories as I shaped them into found poems and as I chose which found poems would be in the book. *Patient Listening* resulted from a prolonged, deep collaboration between the authors/patients I interviewed, their treatment stories, and me. In the process, I was changed. I came to understand what a wise clinician meant when he told me — a very green medical student — that physicians are privileged to hear patients' stories, their secrets, and the most intimate details of their lives.

What Is *Patient Listening*?

Several times while I was creating *Patient Listening*, I sought help from experienced writers and was told, "I'm sorry I can't help you because this isn't poetry. It doesn't rely on images." Another common refrain was "I'm sorry I can't help you because this isn't really prose." Similarly, different readers have had different ideas about the nature of the final product. Given my experience with Anna Deavere Smith's work and Eve Ensler's the *Vagina Monologues* (which came to Iowa while I was working on this book), I called it a performance piece, not really a play but a literary work that is at its best when performed as a series of monologues or as readers' theater. The appellation "performance piece" nevertheless puzzled some readers because this volume doesn't have a dominant story line; it doesn't have a beginning, a middle, or an end. Moreover, these readers felt a performance of the entire piece would be quite long and perhaps overwhelming. They viewed *Patient Listening* more as a collection or anthology of poems or stories.

Why is this question important? I think it is important because "what it is" will affect how it is perceived and, consequently, how it is used. Perhaps the best answer to this question is that *Patient Listening* crosses genres; it doesn't fall neatly into one category or another, which means one is free to use it to suit one's self or one's immediate purpose. One can read, perform, or study it as a whole in which the different characters and poems interact with or comment on each other. I organized the authors/patients to facilitate this reading or use of *Patient Listening*. One could also use it as a collection of poems or stories, reading, savoring, and using small bits at a time. Or one could rearrange the authors'/patients' contributions and found poems, creating new relationships between the stories and the ideas.

Suggestions for How to Use This Book

Health-care educators can incorporate *Patient Listening* into formal or informal teaching sessions in numerous ways. For large group teaching, students or faculty members could present an excerpt as readers' theater during a class period and students could discuss their responses to the piece in small group sessions. (This is the primary way we use *Patient Listening* at the University of Iowa Carver College of Medicine.) A faculty member could present a poem or a short excerpt during a lecture to illustrate a patient's perspective on a specific disease (e.g., Marva Dawn's "Trust Me I'm a Patient" and "It Would Help Me If . . ." for a lecture on diabetes). Students could read *Patient Listening* as background material for a course on doing histories and physical examinations. Faculty members could present *Patient Listening* as readers' theater during retreats, grand rounds, or departmental or divisional meetings. (I have presented *Patient Listening* in this manner for different groups of students, residents, and faculty.)

Likewise, the volume is appropriate for small group teaching. Facilitators could present specific found poems to trigger discussions on topics such as health-care workers' attitudes toward patients with particular characteristics or behaviors. Facilitators could present specific found poems to trigger discussions about ethical issues in patient care such as caring for patients with disabilities, patients who are stigmatized (e.g., who are obese, have used illicit drugs, or are infected with a blood-borne pathogen), patients who are poor and uninsured, patients from other cultures, and health-care workers who become patients. Students could read specific found poems and write reflection papers about two to three things they would do to improve communication with that author/patient. Participants in clinician-patient communication courses or seminars could read or present short excerpts of *Patient Listening* and discuss or practice (e.g., role play) ways to improve communication between the health-care worker and the patient depicted in particular found poems.

Finally, *Patient Listening* is applicable to clinical teaching. Students could create found poems from their patients' histories, or clinical faculty members could read specific poems on rounds or ask their trainees to read specific poems, encouraging them to think about their patients' experiences.

Curriculum Example: Inpatient Clinical Teaching

I field-tested some of these suggestions when I was the attending physician on an inpatient general medical service. I asked my team members to read Dr. Fitzhugh Mullan's found poems. Several days later, I inquired about their responses. After reading the poems, the students noted that the distinction between physicians and patients is a false dichotomy because we are all patients. I also requested that team members create found poems from histories they had obtained from their patients. We all found or wrote poems and then read them out loud to each other. The students and residents were initially timid about sharing their poems but did so enthusiastically after I read mine. Each of them felt that creating the poems had given them more insight into their patients than they had gained through writing the standard medical history. Neither of these "assignments" took my team members much time, nor did the assignments cause them to work beyond the mandatory duty hours.

Curriculum Example: Classroom Teaching

At the University of Iowa Carver College of Medicine, we use the material from *Patient Listening* in a required course for first-year medical students called "Foundations of Clinical Practice I." Selected students present a collection of these found poems as readers' theater for the other students in their class. The grouping that we have found most effective is arranged so that the authors' sections exhibit balance and variety. I specifically chose to start and end with found poems that were centered on the authors' stories in the context of their medical care. In order, the authors and poems most often included in the University of Iowa course are Nancy Mairs ("My Story," "Classic Example," "Teaching Hospital," "Signing On"); Teresa Richards ("Hip Replacements," "Choosing a Doctor"); Richard Selzer ("Night Train," "Tulip Phobia"); Mary Swander ("Open Reduction," "Alternative Route"); Faye Moskowitz ("Checkup," "Telephone Manner"); Arthur Frank ("15-Second Connection," "Drunk Driving," "This Pseudo Thing"); Marva Dawn ("Postdoctoral Training," "Trust Me I'm a Patient," "The Best Medicine," "The Color Red"); Richard Solly ("Assumptions," "Taking Chances," "Tinkering," "Learning to Look"); Laura Evans ("The Wrong Chart," "Living for Mail," "Plastic Hugs"); and Louise DeSalvo ("Self-Prescribing," "A Story to Tell"). Because students have responded well to this arrangement, which can be read during a typical one-hour class period, we have continued to use it in nearly the same form each year.

Several weeks before the performance, a faculty member asks the participating students to read the excerpt and indicate which authors/patients they would prefer to represent. The faculty member then assigns roles to the students based on their preferences. One or two faculty members meet with the readers to practice their roles, coach them on reading the found poems for an audience, and answer questions (e.g., about pronunciation and delivery).

In class, a faculty member briefly introduces the piece (five minutes) and then the students present their parts (between thirty-five and forty minutes). During the remaining class time, all students write responses to the following suggested reflections: (1) Describe at least two things you learned about what it is like to be a patient. (2) Give at least two examples of simple things health-care providers can do to make the health-care experience better for their patients. (3) Which story impressed or affected you most? Describe why you chose this story. Subsequently, students meet in their small groups and discuss their responses to *Patient Listening* and their answers to the reflection questions.

Special Considerations

We have learned from our experience of using *Patient Listening* as readers' theater at the University of Iowa, and at several national and international meetings, that it is helpful to coach the readers on how to read the poems most effectively. We recommend that readers practice reading the poems out loud to work on articulation, pronunciation, and pacing; pause consciously after reading the first-person introduction, each poem title, and each poem; read slowly, in general, and pause briefly before reading important lines, especially those at the ends of poems; change the tone and tenor of their voice (and perhaps their accent) when the poem recounts health-care workers' statements.

We have found that these suggestions help readers counter their natural tendencies to speak too quickly and to drop their voices at the end of statements while reading to an audience. During brief practice periods, inexperienced readers can learn to enunciate clearly and use their voices to emphasize important ideas so that the audience, which usually does not have the text, understands and appreciates the found poems.

Patient Listening enables students to glimpse the experiences and perspectives of patients with whom they have little in common — and, in some cases, for whom they might have antipathy — and thereby develop further their ability to be empathetic caregivers. In some instances, students take on the roles of persons who are radically different from themselves. Female students often read the roles of male patients, and vice versa. Moreover, the students, who are usually young and healthy, portray sick or disabled persons, some of whom are elderly. The differences between the students and the authors/patients whose poems they read can be greater than differences in gender or age. For example, a month after the 9/11 attacks, a Muslim man from a Middle Eastern country volunteered to read the role of Faye Moskowitz, a Jewish woman from the eastern United States, because he enjoyed speaking with different accents.

Responses to *Patient Listening*

In general, the students have received this learning experience very well and have recommended that it remain in the curriculum. A number of comments describe what students learned about the patient's perspective: "Even 'good' doctors can improve their patient care"; "patients appreciate small tokens or gestures that make both them and you more human"; and "physicians must be able to address a wide range of emotions." "Doctors' interactions with patients can significantly affect their state of mind about a disease."

A number of replies are illustrative of students' responses to the question "Which story impressed or affected you most? Describe why you chose this story": "The patient with testicular cancer affected me the most. It showed how simple it is to make all the difference." "The story of the lady with breast cancer who just wanted human touch affected me the most. I didn't think about how important touch is." "The story about Crohn's disease impressed me the most. I could visualize being the patient and not being able to look at my abdomen and I tried to imagine all he went through with the disease." And "The story about the woman with bilateral hip replacements impressed me the most. It just didn't occur to me that cutting out something bad or something causing problems can be emotionally difficult."

My colleagues and I have also surveyed the students who performed the roles of the authors/patients to learn whether these students benefited from their active participation. In general, these students felt that reading their roles helped them "become" their characters and understand the patients' viewpoints better than they previously had. One student said, "Being able to read a poem and be part of the performance was amazing. I actually felt like I knew what my person had gone through. It gave me a new perspective of what being a patient can be like." Another student answered, "It allowed me to try to jump into his head for a moment." One student reflected deeply about identity—her patients' and her own.

> Thank you for the opportunity to portray Marva. When I read her character I connected with her, as my mother has been a diabetic for the past twenty years. In addition, I liked her spunk and attitude about being a person with "bad eyes" and not a blind person. I hope I will always remember this key point; patients are people first, with lives and then with illnesses. I also began to think of the flip side, I will be a person first who happens to be a physician rather than a physician who happens to be a person. While this may sound a little weird, I could foresee myself . . . falling into the machine work of being a physician and losing touch with being a person. This, in turn, may cause me . . . to lose touch with patients as people. This is a concept I need to think out more, but it is a start.

My colleagues Kristi Ferguson and Marcy Rosenbaum and I have identified five major themes in the students' reflections: (1) Illness evokes emotions, and providers must address both the physical and emotional needs of their patients. (2) Patients want health-care providers to listen well and to understand their perspectives. (3) Providers' words and gestures profoundly affect patients. (4) Patients do not want to be defined, identified, or treated as only their symptoms or illnesses. (5) Information and conditions that clinicians consider routine can be very distressing for patients.

The students' comments and our thematic analysis of their comments have led us to conclude that *Patient Listening* helps medical students understand patients' perspectives on health care. This piece also helps students learn that they must listen closely to patients and address them as whole persons.

When we presented an excerpt from *Patient Listening* at a meeting of the Central Group for Educational Affairs, we recruited well-known members of the group to read the roles and we asked the audience and participants to evaluate the piece and suggest ways that it could be used as an educational tool. The responses of both members of the audience and participants corroborated our experience at the University of Iowa. One respondent stated, "Every medical student and doctor should experience this!" and another called it an "incredible teaching tool . . . demonstrat[ing] that the patient's experience is . . . critical . . . to treatment. We miss this in standard teaching. We 'medicalize' everything to protect ourselves from this personal experience."

To further enrich the experience, the audience and participants suggested specific ways that educators could use *Patient Listening*, including during orientation or as a noontime discussion piece for residents. Other participants suggested that students write stories based upon their own interviews with patients or that this approach would be an effective exercise to remind senior medical students of what medicine should be. Additional suggestions included using found poems to trigger discussion in a medical-humanities elective; as the basis for programs in humanism, communication, and the culture of medicine; or formatted as a CD, an audio tape, or a video — and specific discussion questions could be developed for individual vignettes or found poems.

When creating *Patient Listening*, I tried to balance negative and positive poems in the entire piece and in the excerpt that we usually present to medical students and other audiences. Of the ninety-one poems in the book, twenty-eight are positive, fifteen contain both positive and negative, eleven are neutral, and thirty-seven are negative. Despite my efforts, a few people in every audience remember only the negative poems and do not recognize that these critical stories can be redeemed if one listens to them and learns from them. For example, one medical educator responded, "This would clearly be called a 'biased sample.' The writers, in their own self-centered, self-serving ways, [described] self-centered, unfeeling physicians. They are obviously presented for their 'negative shock' value. There are methods to do the same thing which take less time." I can understand this response because as a physician I cringe when I hear the "bad doctor" stories and I hate to have my profession bashed. I did not create this piece to further berate health-care professionals. Rather, I created *Patient Listening* as a tool to help health-care professionals, including myself, hear patients' stories more clearly and respond more empathetically so that both patients and health-care workers will be more satisfied with their interactions. I believe these stories have helped me avoid mistakes and have motivated me to improve the way I relate to patients.

I'm Nancy Mairs.

I've made a career writing personal essays, many of which are about my experiences with illness, of which I have had just a few — allergies, migraine headaches, agoraphobia, depression, and primary progressive MS. I'm quadriplegic but I can still type with my right index finger, two sentences at a time.

My Story

I've looked at my medical record
over the years.
It never feels like me.
It's done in shorthand.
Only one note absolutely
reflected my reality,
moved me, too.

My husband's oncologist
was also my physician.
The note was dated on a day
when I didn't have an appointment.
My husband did.
It had the date and
"Patient is devastated."
I just found out
my husband was dying
of stage IV melanoma.
I was exactly devastated.

But I was moved that this doctor
pulled my records
and wrote something.
He was trying to record
my story
even though it wasn't
my body
that happened to be doing

this particular thing;
it was my soul
that it was happening to.

Classic Example

A psychopharmacologist
I was working with
to find an antidepressant —
I finally fired him —
came in to talk about
the drugs I was taking.
He never looked at me.
He sat on the edge of the sofa,
looking at his lap,
taking notes,
never physically relaxed,
his shoulders rigid.
I laughed and said,
"Have you heard of the great molasses flood?"
He said, "No, but is it pertinent?"
A vat of molasses
in Boston
broke.
Molasses oozed down the street.
A number of people drowned,
horribly.
That's how I feel
when I'm depressed.
So it was
exactly pertinent
but
I couldn't say anything
except, "Yes,
but never mind."

Teaching Hospital

When I go into the hospital
or to a clinic appointment
I go right into
the teaching mode.
I tell them
if they look at my right eye
they ought to see disc pallor,
but if they can't
don't worry
because it's hard to see.
Once nine medical students
in a row
looked at my right eye.
A gang bang.
I thought I'd
never see again.

Signing On

Even neurologists hope.
But they can't hope if you have MS.
No one with MS
ever spontaneously recovered.
It's a whimsical disease.
Nothing they can do.
Well, if you were a doctor
and your ambition was
to make people well,
would you work
with people who could not
be made well
under any circumstances?

My neurologist takes care
of MS people,
on purpose.
She permits us to be ill,
takes good care of us
without requiring us to respond
to her ministrations
by getting well.

We have even talked
about my dying.
She doesn't believe
my death is imminent.
When the time comes,
she will do everything to make sure
it happens comfortably.
She signed on for the duration
in a way
no doctor ever has.

I'm Teresa Richards (a pseudonym). I had
both hips replaced in my late forties and early fifties. I don't have
pain in my hips anymore but my stride isn't normal and I can't do
many of the things I love doing, like running and low-impact aero-
bics. Here's a bit of my story.

Hip Replacements

I remember the day,
   the pre-op eval.
I was furious,
I was going to have this done;
I had made a decision to do it.
I could have stayed,
   limping along.

I remember saying,
   "You have to forgive me,
   I'm mad as hell."
They said,
   "This is going to happen to you."
   "This is what the hips look like."
   "Here's the video."
They sit you in front of a TV.
You watch the video.
They have no clue what happens;
They don't talk
   about the emotional part.

At home, I started thinking.
About those bones, I mean,
   they actually sawed them off,
   threw them away.
Part of my body,
                just thrown away.

Part of me,
                    gone.
Hard to grasp.

I went for the follow-up.
Still agonizing, thinking
    I didn't need hip replacements;
    I could have done something.
Still hanging on to that,
I remember saying to the resident —
    this 16-year-old coming in to take care of me,
    clueless —
"You know the part that takes the longest?
    Emotions."

If somebody drops a line,
like that day I said,
    "I'm mad as hell,"
if somebody just followed up on that,
    then, maybe, they could make it easier.

Choosing a Doctor

I'll tell you a tale.
My wrinkles have gotten worse;
I wanted laser treatment.
I had an appointment;
    this guy was so bad.

Everybody goes to him.
He's great;
    would probably do a great job.
But it was like this wall,
    a masked face just planted there.
He didn't connect with anything I said.
I tried humor;

North York Central Library 416-395-5535

Toronto Public Library

27131018154635

Date Format: DD/MM/YYYY

Number of Items: 2

Item ID:37131095669537
  Title:Patient listening : a doctor's guide
  Date due:18/05/2013

Item ID:37131116732330
  Title:Smith's patient-centered
interviewing : an evidence-based
method
  Date due:18/05/2013

. . .

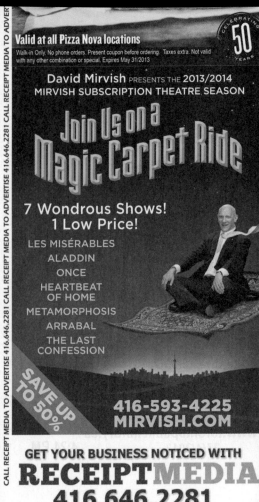

he didn't blink.
Disconnect.

He had his little agenda,
　　his little routine.
He said, "Consultation means learning."
　　Ticked off a list of things;
　　couldn't veer from his script.
He is 50.
Will he change?
No.
　　Could he have thought differently
　　when he was 25 or 30?
Maybe not.

Still,
　　would I have chosen him?
If I had the money?
Probably,
　　because he's good at it.

I'm Richard Selzer.

When I was fifty-eight, I retired from my position as professor of surgery at Yale so I could write full time. Five years later, after a three-week speaking tour, I collapsed in my home from Legionnaire's disease. Twenty-three days later, I woke up in the ICU at my "old hospital." I'd like to share a few of my observations with you.

Night Train

Coma is a deep well.
Gaze into it,
all you see is your own reflection.
I did get the feeling of,
of a kind of velocity,
as though I were on the upper berth
on a Pullman train.
Night,
always night outside.
Nothing to see
except pitch-black night.
Then suddenly there would be
a herd of white-faced cattle.
Then darkness.
Or there would be
a grove of white birch trees.
Then darkness.
Later, it occurred to me
that these moments
were when the nurse or a doctor
lifted my eyelid,
shone a light
to see if my pupils
would constrict or dilate.

Squatters

The hardest part
was the knowledge
that I had surrendered
my body
to strangers
for twenty-three days,
that they knew my body intimately,
in all its particularities,
that I had no say in the matter.
I felt something had been
taken away from me.
My property,
my body,
vandalized.
Somebody else had moved into it,
taken it over,
lived there for a while,
left it in ruins.

Tulip Phobia

When I did recover,
there was a period of insanity.
It happens to people who are
adjuncts to tubes and respirators,
needles and bottles.
I was quite mad.
I had hallucinations,
paranoid thoughts
that lasted weeks.

I was terrified,
clinging to the bed rails
like a parrot to a twig

for fear
the top and the bottom
of the bed
would come together
and I would sink
into this chasm,
be lost forever.
I couldn't see.
I had to hang on,
so
I hung on all night
long.

It was very hard for me
to tell my doctors that
I was afraid of those tulips.
If only someone
would take them away.
I realized
that was crazy.
But as soon as the sun went down,
there they were,
malevolent witches,
their heads
weaving.

In my madness,
I was unreachable.
It was only
when I reached bottom
and there was my nurse, Patrick —
who gave me a bath, and
healed me —
that I could relate
to another human being
who was waiting
for me.

My name is Mary Swander. I had a severe reaction to a bad allergy shot. To cope, I moved to a one-room school house in the Amish area of Iowa, where I grow my own organic vegetables. I have arthritis in my neck after a car accident that broke a cervical vertebra, and I have constant pain from myelitis — a viral infection of my spinal cord. I spend several hours a day caring for my health. In my spare time, I write. I also teach English at Iowa State University.

Open Reduction

In excruciating pain,
   I went to ortho clinic.
A very nice resident
   took my whole history, then
   called the chief surgeon, who
barreled into my room yelling,
   "Show me how you read a book."

So,
   I showed him.

"That's your problem,
   you don't hold it high enough.
That's your whole problem."

Walked out,
   yelling at the resident.

Reduced my neck injury to
   how I held a book.

Alternative Route

People think
  all I do is alternative stuff.
Ironic.

I grew up in the M.D. camp;
Granddad was a country doc.
Chiropractic —
  quackery, bogus.
Osteopathy —
  completely forbidden territory.

Through desperation,
  I took a different route.
I would not be there,
  in the alternative land,
if the M.D. world had anything,
  anything to offer me.
But it doesn't.
  Never did.

Imagine this scene.
Pain clinic,
  1980,
  one bed in the recovery room.
Next to me,
  people with limbs amputated,
  waking from drugged sleep.
Calling out,
"Oh my God, oh
  my God, help me,
  help me, I'm in such pain,
  help me."

Twenty anesthesia residents
  pull the drapes,
  encircle, and
  ask,

"How many times a week do you have sex?"
(A woman moans, "Help me.")
"Oh, I don't know,
  maybe 56, 57,
  I lose track."

They give me 30 nerve blocks;
    really rude,
    rush me through.
Tell me, "Come back in a week."
I say, "That worked for two days."
They get mad.
    "We can't help you.
    Go some place else."

So, I thought
    "Okay, I will go
some place else."

That's the first time
                        I wandered off.

My name is Faye Moskowitz.

I teach in the English Department at George Washington University. My breast cancer was diagnosed by mammogram and treated with lumpectomy and radiation therapy. I never felt sick, just a little tired. I've had some pretty interesting interactions with physicians.

Checkup

I used to go with my mother-in-law
   to her checkups.
Felt the need to sit there with her,
   I suppose, because she couldn't
   maybe she couldn't tell the doctor
   all the things he ought to know.
So she said to him,
   "Doctor, ah, mein cholesterol hurts me."
I thought,
   "Oh, for God's sake,
   your cholesterol hurts you,"
and I started to say,
   "What she means is . . ."
He said, "Faye, let, let her say,
   let her explain what it is."
He didn't laugh,
   didn't think it was funny.
He saw this as some sort of clue
   to what she was experiencing.
And when she would describe,
   in Yiddish, the source of her pain,
he would understand.

Telephone Manner

I had the misfortune
 when the, ah, X-ray came back
 with the shadow on it,
my internist was out of town.
His associate called me,
I had never met her,
 and she was very cold on the telephone.
She called here at work and said,
 "Mrs. Moskowitz,
 have you talked to the X-ray people?"
I said, "No, I haven't, should I have?"
And she said, "Well, yes,
 ah, there was opacity on your X-ray."
So I said, "Wow, whoa."
 This is it,
 I'm dead,
 I'm a dead woman.

She said, "I want you to have an MRI.
I want you to do that right away."
So I said, "OK."
She said, "I will call such and such a place,
I will take care of that for you.
OK, Mrs. Moskowitz?
Goodbye."

I said, "Wait, wait, wait, wait, wait, wait."
She said, "What? What?"
I asked, "What does this mean?
What does an opacity on a chest X-ray mean?"
"It means there is a shadow there.
There is something there that
 ah, that, ah, they don't know,
 they don't know what it is.
So you will have an MRI."

I said, "Well, OK, but you know,
    this is a little frightening to me.
Is there anything else
    you could tell me about that?"

She said, "I will tell you
    that you don't have to worry,
                                    yet."

My name is Arthur Frank. I teach

sociology at the University of Calgary. At thirty-nine, I had a heart attack that my doctors attributed to a viral infection. Fifteen months later, I felt healthy enough to complete a triathlon. But then I noticed a persistent soreness in one of my testicles. Pretty soon, my back was sore too and the pain got so bad I couldn't sleep at night. My doctor misdiagnosed the problem. Months later, a sports-medicine specialist identified the cause — metastatic testicular cancer. I'll tell you a few stories.

15-Second Connection

About 15 seconds
   is all it took.
He looked across
   and said,
"If it's cancer,
   we'll be there with you."
Three seconds; four seconds.

I was lying on the table.
He was palpating.
He said, "There's a mass here."
I asked, "Could it be cancer?"
"If it is,
   we'll be right there with you."

He was.
He wasn't taking care of me,
   but he called when
I was in chemotherapy
   just to see
how I was.

A one-minute phone call.
No medical intervention.

Just wanted me to know
he was concerned,
    still thinking
of me.

Drunk Driving

When these images showed up
    on ultrasound,
the ultrasound guy,
    a prominent physician, said
"It's either primary or secondary tumors.
I'll send a report to your doctor."
Not
    "Good luck," or
    "I wish I could do more for you."

I heard him say
    "You don't have questions.
    I will tell your doctor.
    Take your questions to him.
    Get out of my lab.
    I don't want you here."

Bartenders are
    liable for their customers who
    drink too much and drive.
What about physicians, who
    tell people they have cancer,
    and then
just leave them to drive home?

Manners

It is just manners.
There is nothing complicated about it.
It is just saying
    how does one human being
    relate to another human being.
We don't need complicated frameworks or
    communication stuff.
We just need a moment of thought
    and then
                the decency the situation requires.

This Pseudo Thing

I believed
    when I was really sick
    the system would slow down.
People would pay attention to me.

I found
    exactly the opposite.

When I was really sick,
    I made people much more nervous.
They wanted to leave my room
    much faster.
Medicine became
    truly impersonal.

Not always.
    Obviously, not always.
Not my thoracic surgeon,
    but in a lot of other cases,
    when they would try to be personal,
it was just this pseudo thing.

Before the mediastinoscopy,
   this nurse doing the preop stuff asked,
"How are you and your wife coping?"
"Really, we are doing very badly,
   very badly."
"Well, talk to each other."

She turned and left.

My name is Marva Dawn. I'm a

freelance theologian. As a teenager, I developed diabetes after I had measles. I have some of the complications of diabetes. I'm blind in my right eye and I recently had a kidney transplant. I have neuropathy, which means my nerves don't work right so my GI tract doesn't move properly and I can't feel my feet. Consequently, I shattered my foot and now I'm struggling with recurrent foot ulcers. I've also had an intussusception, breast cancer, jaw problems, and trigger finger. And, oh yes, I'm partially deaf in my left ear.

Postdoctoral Training

I've had to train (chuckling)
a couple of my doctors.
One of my doctors used to give me
endless grief about traveling.
"Why are you going?"
"Doctor, that's my work."
"Why do you have to go?"

Finally one day I said,
"Doctor, does it affect my eyes
to travel?"
"No."
"Well, get one thing straight.
I'm not a blind person.
I'm a theologian
with bad eyes."

I have to keep reminding doctors,
as well as myself,
not to let illness
define me.
It's in attendance, but
it's not all
I am.

He Wouldn't Let It Go

When I had the intussusception,
I got to the hospital in the morning;
  sat around all day.
They couldn't figure out what was going on.
But who suspects intussusception
  in an adult?
Finally, this doctor said,
  "There's something wrong.
  I just don't know what.
  I think we better go in to find out."
At ten o'clock at night,
  they prepped me,
  and did surgery.
The next morning he said,
"Fifteen inches of your bowel
  was crossed over and gangrenous.
You know, if we hadn't gone in
  you'd be dead."

Bless his heart,
that doctor
  just wouldn't rest,
  wouldn't let it go.
It gnawed at him
  and gnawed at him.
He hung around all day
  and just wouldn't let it go.
(pause–crying)

And I'm alive today
as a result.

Trust Me I'm a Patient

People are in too much of a hurry.
I mean, I've never had a major misdiagnosis.
My foot misdiagnosis
    wasn't his fault.
The break didn't show up
    on X-rays.
He didn't investigate more,
    because I was diabetic.
He assumed it was poor circulation.
Told me to walk
    a lot.

So, I've never had major, major —
    you know, people have horror stories
    of misdiagnoses.
I've had lots of cases
    where nurses don't trust me
    to know about my insulin.
What they want to shoot me with
    is going to throw me
    into an insulin reaction.

So, those have been
    bad experiences,
when they haven't trusted me
    to know
            my own body.

It Would Help Me If . . .

It would only take a wee bit,
    a minute
to greet the person and ask about
some joy in their life or
something that's good for them

before you started talking
about all the bad stuff
    so that there was a context
    and the doctor had a broader view
of the patient
    than just the illness.

Patients also need
    answers to their questions.
One of my doctors is always in a hurry
    and I don't always get my questions asked.
Some of them are pretty important.

It would help me if
    the doctor would say,
"What do you
need to talk about
for the sake of fitting
this in with the rest of your life?"

The Best Medicine

I lost my brain on Friday or Saturday.
Got it back Monday.
Tuesday I was let out of the hospital.

The doctor said,
"What are you doing for home care?"
"Doctor, that's something I needed to ask you about."
"Why?"
"I'm going to a speaking engagement tomorrow." (laughing)
"Where?"
"Florida."
"What are you doing?"
"Speaking to pastors and teachers."
"Is it going to be a large crowd?"
"About a thousand."

"You should go."
"Really?"
"Yes, you should go."

That was the best medicine:
    doing what I love,
    doing it well
even though
I was in terrible shape —
25 pounds of extra water
because my kidneys just sort of
stopped working.
    Being with those people,
    using my brain,
    knowing it was working,
was really delightful.
If that doctor hadn't been wise enough to tell me to go —
    isn't that amazing?

The Color Red

A professor noticed his medical students
were just relying on tests,
    not really listening to the patients,
    not really looking at the patients.
They missed a diagnosis that
    would have been obvious
if you just
    looked at the patient,
    really heard the patient.
He made them go to an art museum
    to observe paintings
so they could
    observe patients.
I thought that was the greatest story.
Because, you know,

if you can look at a painting
and see what the person does with color,
you're more likely to notice the coloring
on a wound.
There's a different kind of red
if it's the red for healing
or the red of infection.
Those are two different reds.
But you have to look carefully
to know
the difference.

I'm Richard Solly, a poet, teacher, and editor. I've had Crohn's disease since I was a kid. I had a major episode when I was twenty-five — you know, pain and lots of bleeding. When I was forty, my bowel perforated and I was in the hospital for two and a half months. After that, my abdomen was wide open for one year before they could close the wound. Stories, yeah, I've got stories.

Assumptions

I was experiencing a lot of pain
after surgery.
I mean, for another week
it got worse.
My fever was going up,
I was asking for more morphine.
Some nurses and doctors thought
I was addicted,
I was asking for it more,
and more,
not because I was
in a lot more pain but because —
you know, I was stitched up,
or stapled
and the infection just —
the bowel perforated,
the wound opened,
septicemia,
blood pressure 60/o,
and nobody —
They thought
I was asking for pain medicine
because I wanted it.

Taking Chances

A woman GP said,
"You really went through hell.
How was it?"
An open-ended question.
I said, "Well, it was tough,
still is.
I had some unusual experiences."
It was the first time
I took any chance,
you know,
to say it.
She asked, "What were those experiences?
What do you mean unusual?"
We talked for 45 minutes.
She really helped me
get it focused.
It didn't take much.

You're not asking them
to be a guru,
a Tibetan monk,
a psychologist, or
practice a different field.
Just ask
one more question,
two more questions.
Somehow everything
comes into place
much quicker.

Tinkering

I cut class;
saw Mary Swander,
talked for two,
two and a half hours.
We laughed,
joking, poking fun
at medical people
for our benefit,
at their expense.
You do that.
On the other hand,
my surgeons and doctors —
I'd be dead
if it weren't for them.
So, I owe them my life,
but I don't owe them all,
I don't owe them everything (laughing).

I really have had good doctors.
They've been great.
On the other hand,
I think they're robbing —
it's hard to say this to you —
but I think they're quacks (laughing).
You know,
they're all guessing.
They're like mechanics.
"Well, I really don't know
what this is,
but we'll tinker around
and see."

They're making an incision
up your abdomen,
working on your intestines.

This is not your intestines
they're working on,
this is who you are,
your body
and soul.

Learning to Look

I used to pull the sheet up
and my gown
because I didn't want to look,
didn't think I needed to.
I was in the hospital;
they were taking care of my wound.
I didn't want to glimpse
this huge area of red tissue —
oh my God,
that wasn't supposed to be there.
I didn't want to look.
Who would?
So I would struggle to pull that gown
over my face.

The nurses irrigated the wound,
cleaned it,
changed the bandages.
Gruesome.
They all did it right.
But one nurse saw me
struggling,
gave me a towel.
She understood,
helped me accomplish
what I wanted.
After that I didn't need a towel anymore,
didn't need to cover up.

It was like, man,
this is getting a little much.
I looked at the ceiling,
slowly started looking
at it.

I'm Laura Evans.

In August of 1989, just after I turned forty, I discovered a lump in one of my breasts. My mammogram was negative so my doctor didn't think it was anything to worry about. I believed him. Three months later while on a business trip in South Korea, I felt a lump in my armpit. I was diagnosed with stage III breast cancer and I went through a bone-marrow transplant when they were still experimental procedures. In 1995, I was the first person who had had a bone-marrow transplant to climb a major peak — Aconcagua at 22,841 feet, in Argentina. I've had some good and some bad experiences with medical people.

The Wrong Chart

A doctor in Boise,
the first oncologist I went to meet with,
kept me waiting for half an hour.
I was horrified.
He called me by the wrong name.
I mean, you are overly sensitive
when you are going through this
because you think,
"Well, my life is in the balance here,"
and you want somebody —
you want their full attention.
You don't want to think that maybe
they picked up the wrong chart,
or they don't really care.
Then, he just kind of said
"This is what I recommend.
We can hook you up right now."
And I'm like "Well, I don't think so."
He seemed to be in a real hurry
to just hook me up.
So I never went back to him.

Living for Mail

There was a nurse who was jealous of me.
Don't you love that?
I mean, I'm in there dying.
Everything had to be sterilized,
and I lived for my cards.
She wouldn't sterilize them until like late in the day.
She said,
"Oh, yeah, you got mail,
I just haven't gotten around to getting them sterilized.
I haven't gotten around to it."
I mean, I lived for that.
That was sad.
She was, I don't know —

Plastic Hugs

There were plastic sleeves
that came in to my bubble.
When I was really sad
a couple of nurses would give me hugs.
I loved that.
Like, "Thank you."
You know,
I was with no human contact (tearful).
Every little bit helped.
So, that made a difference.

I'm Jane Smiley.

I'm a writer, teacher, and horse-woman. Several years ago, I had kind of a freak accident. I fell off my horse; the ground was hard and my heel came down last, like a hip whiplash. I saw my heel hit and I knew I had broken my leg.

Every time the orthopedist tried to describe what he had done or what my injury was, I would faint. Yeah (laughing), I didn't want to hear it because I didn't want to know what the challenge was. I just focused on the idea that it was a passing thing. The tibia had a fracture but the fibula was kind of smashed. And I didn't understand why I needed a fibula in the first place. So, I probably took what some people would consider a frivolous attitude towards it, but I decided that was the way to deal with it.

Whose Illness Is It Anyway?

First, let me say that
healing is kind of organic and
fixing is kind of mechanical.
The surgeon was of the fixing mode.
That was just fine
for this particular issue.

My orthopedist
had a kind of breezy, arrogant manner, and
he was young,
probably only about 35.
He was always telling me what a great job he did
putting my leg together,
you know, and having me acknowledge
that he was a great surgeon.
I didn't want to focus on what a great job he did or
the extent of the injury, or whatever.
I thought he was into the surgery
as his personal experience (laughing)
rather than mine.

And I just thought that was
sort of inappropriate.
I think there is always a disparity between
how the patient feels and
the way the doctor feels
about something that is going on.

There are two things going on
whenever you and your patient are in your office,
and they are not exactly similar.
One is your experience of the creativity,
the fascination, and the pleasure
of this illness as an intellectual challenge,
and maybe as a personal challenge.
And the other is the spiritual and physical transition
of the patient as he is coming to terms with his condition
and trying to, you know, overcome it or
accommodate it, or whatever.
I think the patient is insulted and offended
if he feels that the physician's experience
is more primary to the physician than
the patient's experience.
Do you see what I mean?
I think it is a challenge for physicians,
because to participate in the patient's experience
means being vulnerable to that human side.
And the illness might be so interesting that in some sense
you can't contain your glee (chuckling).
So, I think that's a fine line that physicians
have to walk.

I am Michael Gearin-Tosh,

an Oxford don who teaches English. I've also been a theater director and I'm currently involved in haute couture. About nine years
ago, I was diagnosed with multiple myeloma. The doctors I saw,
talked with, corresponded with, or with whom my friends talked
and corresponded, gave conflicting advice. Some said I had to have
chemotherapy immediately or I was going to die. Others said if I
touched chemotherapy I was a dead man. Ultimately, I sided with
the latter and did a modified Gerson therapy — no meat or salt, lots
of raw vegetables and fruit, lots of juices, B-12 injections, and coffee
enemas — with Chinese breathing exercises and visualization. So
far I've beaten all the odds. Let me share a few of my observations
with you.

Physician-Assisted Suicide

Anemia is partially a blessing
if you are very ill
because it turns you down.
I didn't have the energy to be hysterical.
I just took it
one day at a time.
What else can you do?

I thought that if I had to die
I would rather die
18 months earlier
than to be put through a bone marrow transplant,
this thankless dying process,
which was going to be
absolutely ghastly.
And we all have to die.
So why not just die?

If you take that
from the standpoint of somebody
who is well and energetic,
they might take
a different point of view.
When you are very anemic
and exhausted
it's not such a huge deal
if you go to sleep
and don't wake up.

One cancer specialist
actually said to me —
it's not just my imagination —
that if he had my cancer
he would commit suicide.
It made me think,
though this seems a very glib rationalization,
that his treatments were
close to people committing suicide
without agreeing
to it.

Evidence-Based Medicine!

Oh God, have I heard about it.
Have I thought about it.
It's one of these extraordinary
medical misnomers.
I mean, what is evidence-based medicine?
I think it tends to mean that
if you have a double-blind trial
you will establish something called
evidence.
It seems to me
very important to define

what is the nature
of that evidence.

Let me tell you about a double-blind trial
done or tried to be done
on part of the Gerson diet by Professor Cornell.
I mean, this is a real life case.
He thought he would do a double-blind trial
on carrot juice.
Well, you can't do a double-blind trial
with more than one factor at a time.
So you get 10 patients
who get carrot juice
and you get another 10 patients
who think they are getting carrot juice,
but they are not.
And you compare the results over 2 years.
That would be an evidence-based trial
which would produce
something called evidence.
Well, of course,
they quickly ran into the problem
of how you create a substitute
for fresh carrot juice.
You can't.
After a few days of watery gluck
or a few hours,
the placebo people said,
"This isn't fresh carrot juice."
So they said, "Oh fine,
we can't do it this way.
What we will have is beta-carotene capsules."
So they did the trial with
beta-carotene capsules.
Well, I don't have to tell you
that biochemical knowledge

is not sufficiently advanced
to detect what might be in carrot juice
but is not in a beta-carotene capsule.
The likelihood is that there's a very great deal
that is in fresh carrot juice
that is not in the capsule.
Collapse of the trial.

This simply points to the wider issue
that of course you have to see
if you can establish evidence for efficacy.
But the danger is that when you get
something called evidence
you think it's
hard, conclusive evidence
and that's the last thing it is.
To begin with,
the very difference between human beings
would suggest limitations
to the evidence.
Even if the capsules did work,
suppose all 10 who got the capsules did better
than the 10 who got placebos.
I would want to know the percentage of depressives
among the placebos
who weren't going to do well anyway.
But then suppose you wanted to do
evidence-based trials on what I do.
Carrot juice,
lettuce juice,
wheat grass juice,
breathing exercises followed by visualizations,
shots of vitamin B-12,
food without salt,
no fried food,
expeller-processed flax oil.

You couldn't begin to do it.
All of it would take you a lifetime.

Cancer is a disease
which is imperfectly understood.
When you are dealing with uncertainty
you have to remain cautious
about what you conclude.

Cancer Doctors

Doctors are only human.
A very mixed bag I assume.
Cancer doctors are among the heroes
of the modern world.
But they are in a terrible
terrible position.
They're dealing with a horrible disease
which is imperfectly understood.
They're overworked;
there are far too few of them.
Their patients are in a highly agitated state;
they haven't time to get to know them.

When you get a disease like cancer,
you are asking from doctors
a very rare combination of two things
which don't obviously go together.
You want doctors to be trained
so that if you break your legs
you get someone
who knows what to do with a broken leg.
That's very different from
what you do or don't do with a fatal disease
which you don't understand,
which operates differently
in each of your patients.

I'm Emily Douglas (a pseudonym). My medical history started early — I was born with erythroblastosis fetalis, which meant my mother made antibodies against my blood type, causing my blood cells to break apart or hemolyze. I had lots of transfusions to get me through until the hemolysis stopped. As my mother put it in her stoic fashion, "You were sick for several months and then you were cured." When I was twenty-two, I struggled with anorexia, which I overcame only to be diagnosed eight years later with Chronic Fatigue Syndrome and environmental allergies. Suddenly I was dragged into a dizzying exhaustion. I was allergic to everything from mold to perfume, from wheat to ragweed. I've spent a lot of time trying to find the right doctors.

Intuitive Trust

The worst period of time was when
I was so fatigued I couldn't get up off the couch —
I tried all the old remedies
    and the rituals I'd done before
    and I just never got better.
I finally got up,
    called the Academy for Environmental Medicine,
    and asked for a listing of people in my region.
They gave me the name of a doctor in Atlanta.
He was an M.D. I wanted an M.D.
I didn't want to do the Yellow Page thing.
Atlanta was five hours away and I was really exhausted.
I didn't know how I was going to make the trip.
I didn't know if I could stay awake.
But I went.

When I saw the doctor,
    he looked at me.
He looked at my toenails.
He looked in my eyes.

He looked at my skin
    at its color and texture.
He looked at me in a different way
    than most people had been looking at me.

I immediately trusted him.
I cannot give you any reason for that.
It was just intuitive.
    I trusted his intuition;
    I trusted his rigor;
    I trusted his base of knowledge.

He ran a lot of tests,
    tests for Epstein Barr,
    all kinds of blood counts,
    the traditional tests as well.
He did the IV for me himself
and he stayed there — a witness — watching it drip.
He did that every visit.
    That made a difference to me.
    That calmed me.

Plus, he insisted that I be extremely restrictive.
He gave me a routine.
    It's like doing homework. You know,
    I felt good because I could check it off.
He gave me a narrative that I had to live by
and he made it real clear that this was not going to be
    simple and easy
and it was not going to be
  a magic bullet
                    at all.
It was going to be slow and steady.
    I had to be rigorous.

If you have my kind of personality,
    you love that.
You just go, "Oh, thank you,"

because rigor makes you feel successful.
It's gratifying for patients
    to know that there is a structure,
    some sense of control
because you feel out of control
    with anything that is episodic and chronic.

But I guess more than anything,
    he gave me hope.

Making a List

I always make a list.
I mean, I always go prepared
    to a doctor's appointment.
I always go with very specific questions
    and very specific issues
hoping that we will cover them
    and that the doctor will ask me things
I haven't come up with myself.
The thing is,
    you really want to please your doctor,
    you want to be such a good pupil.
It is utterly bizarre to me that you go in
    and you think
I'm taking up your time, but
    of course I'm paying you.
I'm taking up your time, and
    I want to make it worthwhile.

The Whole Truth

In terms of the patient's narrative,
             as opposed to the tests —

Listen to both.
It has got to be both.

Both have a level of truth;
             neither of them have the whole truth.

Usually.

Hard to Hear

Suffering is particular,
and personal,
and private.
And it's very hard to hear
the narrative
of suffering.

I'm Steve Kuusisto.

In March 1955, I was born three months early. I was left with retinopathy of prematurity. Even though I was legally blind, my parents gave me a bike and sent me to public schools. I was blind, but I didn't know how to be a blind person, how to travel securely through the world. Instead, I kept making my world smaller and smaller so I could cope.

When I was thirty-nine, I finally got Corky, my first guiding-eye dog. I discovered that I could go places and I had freedom. I later became the director of students for Guiding Eyes for the Blind, the school that trained Corky and me. Now I teach courses in creative nonfiction at the University of Iowa and serve as a public humanities scholar in the University of Iowa's College of Medicine. I also write poetry and nonfiction, and do consulting on disabilities.

Eye Doctors I Have Known

I have to say
most of the eye doctors I have met
have been very cold, clinical people,
who snap those lights on,
look into the back of your skull,
write down the numbers, and
have very little to say.
So, I've seldom had a good experience
with an eye doctor.
It isn't to say that I haven't had one;
I've just seldom had one.

When I was in graduate school,
I went in to see an ophthalmologist for a checkup.
In the middle of the examination,
he went out of the room
without telling me what he was doing,
and he came back in with another physician.
He began talking about me in the third person.

"You're going to encounter people like this
when you go out into practice.
Hey, by the way,
where are you going to practice?
Have you decided yet?"

Later, I went to a retina specialist,
who was highly recommended to me.
He made me wait two hours.
The great man came in
and began talking to me
very quickly.
He walked out of the room
and went across the hall to see another patient.
Then came back in
and talked to me for a few more minutes.
He walked out of the room again.
He was seeing six patients
at once.
And he never had a satisfactory conversation
with me
about my eye condition.
I finally stood up
and I walked out.
I said to the staff, "I'm not paying for this.
I will find a physician that actually imagines
I'm a real person,
and a meaningful patient.
Thanks very much."

My sister is a physician in New York.
She would probably say,
"Yeah, yeah.
They treat everybody like shit.
What makes you think you're so special?"

The best eye doctor that I ever saw
took an interest in the patient.
She took time to ask questions.
What has your experience of blindness been like?
What can you do?
What would you like to do?
What are you interested in?
How does lighting affect you?
Can you hold your eye still
long enough to use this particular device,
or to look through a telescope?

She tried to figure out what could assist the patient.
She was helpful.
Not only did I feel that my situation
was being dignified,
but out of that came some ideas
about adaptive approaches I might take.
She did a slow, thoughtful analysis of who I was,
what might be good for me.

Disability Disconnect

Disability is
                    the enemy.
Disability is
                    the de facto admission of defeat,
the admission that medical practice
                    has failed.
This has a great deal to do with pedagogy,
    how medicine is taught.
Doctors aren't trained in thinking
    about you as a whole being.
Right?
    Why, that would be hand holding,
    wouldn't it?

That's somebody else's job.
This seems to me to be a profound mistake.

What is a quality life?
Who gets to decide?
That of course is the crux of the biscuit —
as my grandpa would say —
that is the crux of the biscuit
with the medical doctor
                    who can't talk to a disabled patient.
That doctor has decided this life
                    can't be valuable,
                    can't be interesting,
                    can't be full, or rich, or what have you.
And silence transmits a great deal.

There is a huge   disconnect
that comes when doctors find
they have reached the end of their efficacy
when treating patients they probably can't cure.
    "You're going to be blind.
    I've reached the end of my magic
    as an ophthalmologist."
    "Your hearing loss is complete."
    "The rehab experience has come to an end."

The patient is either
                    fixable or not.
And if the patient isn't fixable,
    many physicians don't want to go further.
Most eye doctors look at the blind person and say,

"Can't be fixed."

I am Christina Middlebrook.

In the summer of 1991, I was diagnosed with metastatic breast cancer. I went through conventional chemotherapy and then on February 1, 1993, I had a peripheral stem-cell transplant. I had been a healthy person all of my life and I became very, very ill very quickly, as one does with cancer treatments when you've had no symptoms from the cancer itself. I was forty-nine years old. I was raising a family. I had a full-time professional career as a Jungian psychotherapist, and suddenly I became only a cancer patient dying, going through horrendous treatments. I didn't know who I was. My identity was lost. Writing helped me know I was the same person I was before I started cancer treatment. When I was first ill, I made a note in my journal that the irony was I wasn't going to write about it because it was too overwhelming to the brain. But things would happen that I just had to write down because they were so profound for me. As I said in my book, it is hard to remember being killed — yes, that's what the transplant felt like. But in the years since the transplant, memories about my care have returned.

Look at Me

I had a couple of bad experiences.
The worst was when I was in radiation.
I was getting esophageal damage
from the radiation on my vertebrae.
I couldn't get their attention.
No radiation oncologist ever looked in my mouth.
I had a terrific case of thrush.
I couldn't swallow a sip of water
and I couldn't eat.
They treated it symptomatically.
When I told my surgeon
I was losing weight
and I was dehydrated,

she said, "Let me see."
Then she said, "My God!"
and prescribed a medication
to treat a fungus infection
thriving in my throat.
I still have permanent damage.

I thought that was atrocious.
Terrible.
They forgot to look at me.
They were just looking at my slides —
not my slides, my pictures.
That was the worst.

Life Can't Be Fixed

I wish all doctors could be ill,
                              because life can't be fixed.
We aren't going to have lives where
        we don't get ill;
        we don't have unexpected losses.
You just have to give up and surrender.
Surrender is a good word.

I think some doctors are understandably
        so hell-bent on fixing
that they don't know how to
        stay with the unfixable and know how healing,
        as opposed to curative,
it might be to just stay with people
in these impossible dilemmas of
    You might not get better
        and this is all you've got.
    Your life now is living with something
        you never expected.
Life isn't just feeling good and being happy.

Sometimes life is a long time of living
    with something very compromising
            that can't be fixed.

It is very existential.

Witness

When you are sick,
people are encouraging you to get better
and you don't think you're going to get better.
    You feel like a failure.
    You feel better not talking about it. So,
    you just take it inside, and
    you are lonely.
If you have someone there —
a nurse, a doctor, a friend, or a family member —
who can acknowledge that you're getting worse
and how bad that feels
without saying you are going to get worse forever,
    or that you should be getting better,
    or that the woman in the next room is getting better,
    or that somebody else died,
but just stay with you and witness where you are,
you feel
    much less lonely,
        much more connected.
You feel met.
I think it is easier to come back
and not be permanently damaged from the trauma
when you know there is a place
that accepts you as you are.
It keeps the bridge open.

I can't remember what I would say
to the nurses in the middle of the night

when I was so ill.
They didn't try to cheer me up.
One of them, I remember her so well,
her name was Holly;
she was just a student.
She sat with me in the middle of the night and talked.
I was worried about going home,
worried about the treatment.
Was it going to work?
She didn't correct me or say, "Don't worry."
It was wonderful.
She was just a student.
I've always wondered if I could find her again.

The Right Lingo

I also had a doctor,
who I stopped going to,
who was always being upbeat and cheery.
I couldn't tolerate that.
He was making me feel lonely and unlistened to.

When my bone-marrow-transplant doctor was giving me
severe statistics about metastatic disease,
he looked up at me and said,
"Am I being too harsh?"
I said to him, "That's right for me,
that's the way I need to go, I'd like to hear that."
But the upbeat doctor
couldn't hear what I tried to say.
I would have very low white counts.
I really was struggling and he'd say (loudly)
"Oh, it's not quantity, it's quality.
You are really a feisty lady and you'll make it!"
I couldn't find the right lingo

to say to him that that didn't help me.
I wanted him to know that when my white count
wasn't even 3,000, I felt rotten.
And he was making me feel like I, you know,
I should just be smiling and go on with it.
I couldn't get through.

You Can't Do Everything

I sometimes felt the doctors were hurried;
    yes, sometimes.
But that happened while I was recovering
    and doing well.
The sicker people got more attention.
I don't need as much of their time as I used to.
But when I was really sick,
    I felt I got it.

I don't think you can ask your doctor
                                to do everything.
Everyone, I'm sure, is disappointed in their doctor.
                        It's too large a job.
My doctor disappointed me at times.
But, man, was he ever there for me
                        when it counted.

I just wish —
    well, I wish he paid more attention to my pain.
When the problems I had
    weren't related to cancer,
    he wasn't interested.
I had a lot of shortness of breath;
    he referred me to a pulmonologist.
I needed an exercise program
    geared toward women
    who couldn't even touch their toes.

He tried to treat the pain and stamina problems medically
and they weren't medical issues.

It was his staff—
I was walking out with a prescription for a fentanyl patch
and one of the nurses said,
"Oh, my God, you don't know how to handle this.
Why don't you go to the pain clinic?"
I had no idea such a thing existed.
My doctor should have told me,
"This isn't a medical problem anymore.
Why don't you go to the pain clinic?"
It never, in three years of discussing,
it never came up.

And sexuality—
It wasn't just pain with intercourse,
I had no libido.
My gynecologist and my oncologist tried to help
and I'm grateful to them.
Time takes care of it, but they didn't know that.
No one could tell me that.
All they could do was prescribe testosterone,
which is helpful, and vaginal lubricants.

My oncologist said it was amazing to him
to see how important
sexuality remained
in the face of death.

I love that phrase.

A Real Person

One of the things they did at the hospital —
  which I thought was wonderful —
they suggested that we bring a picture of ourselves
  from our healthy days
  and put it in the corridor
so that whoever went in from, what I call, the healthy side,
  could recognize that two months ago
this is what I looked like
  even though I looked like a skeleton,
                    bald, bloated,
      a relic in the bed.

I thought that was wonderful
because it reminded
not the people who work there every day
  but the nutritionist,
  and the lab techs,
  and the other people who came in
that this is a real person in this bed,
  and this is what she looked like just two months ago,
  and this is what she will look like again.
Because you do look so awful
when you have had a bone marrow transplant.

The Other Side

A very prominent oncologist once said to me,
  "I haven't read your book
  because I didn't feel I needed to."
I kind of gulped and thought,
  "Oh lord, one of those."
We went on talking.
Later he said,
  "I think I will read it."

But I was offended.

I was offended that he would feel
    that seeing it from   the other side,
he would know what it was like
    to be going through it

        in the bed.

Shoulder Hugs

My doctor puts an arm around me
whenever he sees me.
That has always felt wonderful to me.
I'm sure someone told him
to touch his patients.
He puts his arm around me from the side
just like a father
putting his arm around his daughter
on the sidelines of her soccer game.
He doesn't embrace me.
He doesn't caress me.
When he came to the bone-marrow-transplant unit,
he would touch my forearm
when he talked to me.
It is helpful.
You think this doctor really cares about you.

One day after an office visit
when he was leaving he said,
"Oh, I haven't touched you."
He came around and gave me
that arm around the shoulder hug.
I thought, "You've got it.
I bet someone taught you to do that."

I am Oliver Sacks, a neurologist and writer.

On Saturday, August 24, 1974, I was hiking by myself on a 6,000-foot mountain in Norway. As I was nearing the top, I walked out of some mist, around a boulder, and saw a bull. As I rushed down the steep, wet path, I fell and tore my left quadriceps tendon off my patella. I tied my leg to my umbrella with strips that I tore from my jacket and scooted down the mountain, using my arms to push my body forward and my right leg to steer. After seven hours, I was nowhere near civilization. I thought I was going to die. But reindeer hunters, who heard me clattering over the rocks, rescued me and got me to a hospital. Febrile and delirious, I was evacuated to London. When I came to after the surgeons reattached the tendon, I thought that the worst had happened, the melodrama was over. I would be fine.

But when I tried to tense my quadriceps muscle, it wouldn't move. The muscle was limp, atonic; it felt like jelly or cheese. I had no sense of where the leg was in space. It was attached to me but it seemed to be an unrelated object. It wasn't mine. Physical therapy didn't help. My knowledge of neurology didn't help. My surgeon told me it was nonsense. My leg was fine; he had fixed it. The registrar told me they had done the necessary carpentry work and he had never heard of anything like this. He was, as he said, a practical man who had no time for listening to my experience and it wasn't his problem that the leg he fixed didn't work. I had hoped my doctors would reassure me, would help me understand what was happening. Instead, by telling me nothing was wrong, they took away my foothold on reality, so to speak. I felt like I was in Limbo.

Alienation

So, it was this strange feeling
of something, which is maybe
quite common, or not that uncommon,
but oddly difficult to express and talk about.
I got a sort of horror from the alienation,

an uncanny feeling, an unearthly feeling.
It shook all my categories.
I didn't know what had gone on.
It certainly disturbed me
not being able to communicate it.
It didn't help that the surgeon said
there was nothing going on.
I even said to myself,
"Don't be silly, Sacks.
You've never heard of anything like this.
A lot of nonsense.
Buck up. Grow up.
You have no time for this."

I like to document and
establish the reality of something.
But if it is something so subjective,
how does one do so?
It was not just communication denied,
it was the reality of my own experience being denied.
There was no one to whom I could talk
in a patient-physician way,
someone who might have
known me well enough
to validate this.

Fear and passivity,
    abjection and subjection,
can go with illness.
It is very complex because one may need to be carried,
    taken care of,
and yet —
    there mustn't be too much
    submission, or
    subjugation, or
    whatever.

I found this especially unpleasant in the hospital
    because I felt I was submitting
to someone who was denying
    my experience.

Hysteria

I wondered if I was hysterical,
    and, indeed,
I hoped I might be.

A psychiatrist came to see me.
He looked at me very carefully
    and said, "This does not have
    the quality of dissociation."
He thought there was
    some organic disconnection,
    but, mostly, he thought I might be obsessing.

I certainly was obsessed by it,

                    this ghostly bloody thing.
So, that both pleased and displeased me.
Better to be mad
    than a cripple.
I feared being
    permanently disabled,
even at one point thinking,
    I would be better off without

                    this ghostly bloody thing.

Uneventful Recovery

I did, in fact,
    steal a look in my own chart
    when I was in the convalescent home.

I saw that the tumultuous events
  of six weeks or whatever
  had been condensed
  to two words, which were
"Uneventful recovery."

A Feeling for the Organism

The good doctor has to be curious
  and he has to be concerned.
If he is curious without being concerned,
  he could become a sort of Nazi doctor,
  or a frenetic investigator,
  or an evangelist.

On the other hand, concern alone
  is slushy and sentimental.
One has to have a strong notion
  and a strong desire to know the particular
    anatomical,
        physiological,
            pathological processes
that are going on
and at the same time
  be attentive to the patients,
    how old they are,
        all their contexts, and
            how they deal with things.

A good doctor ought to be quite intuitive
  and try to hear or sense
    what lies behind the words or complaints.
I would use that McClintock phrase of
  "a feeling for the organism" —
    the equivalent of a green thumb,

which is sort of a feeling or smell
for what is going on.

As a neurologist, I see
much that is incurable and terrible.
On the other hand,
there is almost always something to be done.
I may not be able to reverse a disease,
but whatever it is,
there will be something.

My name is Richard McCann.

I have a Ph.D. in English from the University of Iowa and I co-direct the creative writing program at American University in Washington D.C. I've published several books of poetry and of short stories and my work has appeared in prestigious journals and anthologies. But sometimes it seems as if my biggest story is the one I'm in, the one called "Hepatitis C and Richard McCann's Liver: His Own and the Transplanted Liver." I feel, at times, that I don't want to get near you doctors because you're going to tell me stuff. I'd rather just go with how I'm feeling right now. I also wish doctors would listen to me tell my story in my own way, in my own language.

Stamped

Having hepatitis C
always embarrassed me.
Before my very first biopsy,
I had to give a medical history
and when I was done
the intake nurse got this big red stamp —
to my mind it was 3 feet by 4 feet —
but it couldn't have been because
the size of the file is 8 inches by 14 inches.
She took this big stamp,
and stamped
IVDU
across the front of my file,
stamped it on my intake page.
I thought, Oh my God!
Ya know, I shot drugs three times in college,
and from this moment on
I'm not going to be a professor anymore.
I'm not going to be a person
with as much education

as everyone in here.
I'm not going to be anybody.
I'm going to be
IVDU.

My Primary Care Physician

One of the reasons
I love my primary care physician,
one of the reasons I chose her,
is that before she went to medical school,
she was a book review editor.
I had read some of her reviews
and I thought,
Okay.

When I got sick,
when I was put on the transplant list,
it was clear I had entered a new realm
with my primary care physician,
the home phone number, and all that.
And that meant the world to me.
The seven years since my transplant
have hardly been problem free.
I've called her from foreign countries having problems.
She doesn't just say
"Why don't you go to the ER?"
I fractured my leg in the Virgin Islands,
and it was just a bad situation to be in.
I was calling her everyday,
she was telling me exactly what to do
and what not to do.
The whole time she has taught me,
she's taught me how to take care of myself.
She prepared me, equipped me
to be alone in the world,

to be out living,
and when things happen
I'm not completely in the dark.

I'm going to sing her praise
in another way.
I've gotten no grief from her
about self-medicating.
None.
I tell her everything I do,
I tell her some things in retrospect.
She never gets on my case.
She corrects me sometimes,
she tells me why something I want to do
is a bad idea,
but she never gets on my case
about the fact that
I have taken charge.

When I was in the hospital,
after my first esophageal bleed,
I was in there for a long time.
It was not a hospital she was affiliated with.
She was not in charge of my case.
Anyway, she would come out there periodically.
I was in this horrible shared room,
and there was no place to sit.
She would sit on the floor next to my bed
and talk to me.
I loved her for it.

My primary care physician
is someone I dearly love;
even if she sometimes drives me insane
with her psychologizing,
she's a terrific doctor.
There's no hurrying in and out.

She wants your whole person there,
and she's willing to be there too.

Why Patients Can't Talk to Doctors

You don't say what you feel
to the man you've married
for money.
You say what you feel
to the one you've married
for love.
The dependency is so great,
patients can't risk much.
Do you know what I mean?

I don't think doctors know
how strong the dependency is.
Or, maybe they do,
and it must be very frightening.
Is it?
It must be.

You doctors —
not all of you —
but a lot of you are really smart.
And, I like that, I really like it.
And, if you're not,
okay, I'll go someplace else.
But I feel like, no matter what I do,
I'll never be smart to you.
No matter what I do.
I can write about it.
I can give you copies of stuff
I have written about it.
You will take no interest.
That is very disappointing to me.

No doctor, except
my own primary care physician,
has ever said to me,
"You've learned a lot."
My primary care physician once asked me,
"What do you think is going on here?
You've learned a lot more than I have
about hepatology in recent years."
That meant a lot.

I'd also like the doctor to express
astonishment.
The doctor could say,
"You really care about your situation,
don't you?
I see how important this is to you.
Let me rise to it."

Maneuvering

It's the old thing, you know.
Black people always know white people
    better than whites know blacks.
Your maid always knows you far more than
    you know her.
Your patients spend a hell of a lot of time trying to
        figure you out,
            maneuver around,
                make sure they get what they need.
You don't spend the same amount of time
    on the same issues;
you spend it diagnostically, of course,
    and on treatment.
Or when you have a problem patient, you think,
    how do I get him to be compliant?

But that's a different thing
        than having to figure out
            how to get what you want.
It's a different thing than
        "You better be compliant."

My Body, My Story

Because I'm doing pretty well,
    my hepatology appointments
    are nonphysical.
They are all blood work and chat.
When your liver function is going down,
    there is a lot of checking for
    broken veins,
        how much muscle tissue you're losing, and
        you know, ascites.
You are palpated regularly
    for liver size and everything.
That's the only way I like my story
    in relation to the doctor's office.
I like the numbers of course,
    but I'd like to say to the doctor
Okay —
    I'll listen to it.
    I'll listen to the truth.
    I'll hear everything,
        but in exchange
    I get to lie down
        and you palpate.

I don't know why that means so much to me —
    to be touched of course.
And also because that's the difference between
    one kind of story and
    another kind of story.

I come in with my body
    that's the story I've been dragging
    around with me all this time.
It's got a lot of problems.
    Hydroseal from ascities,
    broken veins up and down
        my lower extremities.
The stuff from portal hypertension,
    it's all there.

I know a doctor can look at me and go
Oh, uh-huh.
    Some gynecomastia,
    probably liver disease.
It's shameful to me, some of the things
    that have happened to my body.
But still it's mine.
    It's my story, the whole damn thing.

I've learned to read your story.
I have a lot of education,
and I know what that means to you.
I'm a relief
    because you can use your lingo with me.
I'm a pain in the ass
    for the same reason.
I know I'm going to have to earn your attention
    by making myself
            of personal interest.

 If you want to say to me,
"I'm happy with the albumin."
 I'll go,
"Me too."
 Maybe for you, this is a nice moment
 because the other guy will go,
"What's albumin?" or
"Huh?"

I've demonstrated how much I respect you.
I've learned your language
   as much as possible.
Sometimes, I misuse it,
   which you like,
     because then you get to correct me.
And it reminds you of who you are.

I've gone to a lot of trouble,
   to learn how to read those lab tests.
I've been to educational seminars
   and I've done a lot of reading.
I can read medical journals.
I couldn't do that before.
I've stretched, and stretched, and stretched.

What I need sometimes is part of my story
   and my language to be spoken.
As it turns out —
ah, it makes me cry to say it —
   my language is my body.
Touch me.
   I don't expect you to hug me.
When you tell me I'm really, really sick,
   I do expect you to touch my shoulder briefly.
I want you to say,
"Mr. McCann, take your shirt off,
   lie down, let me see."
Tick tock tick tock.
And I want you to tell me
   when you hear those sounds.
I want to learn
   what you're hearing,
because what you're hearing is me.
It's me.

You don't know that I'm speaking
   another language

the whole time, the whole time.
It's not that you have to speak it.
One of us is in a foreign country,
    and I think it's me.
I'm your Spanish cleaning lady.
And we spend a lot of time,
    me figuring what you mean,
    what you're saying.
"This is how you run the dryer,"
    because I don't speak so good.
And it touches me when you say, at the end,
"Gracias."
And bend a little my way,
    you know?
It just brings me back in the room a bit.
I'm worthy of being invoked.

So, that's what I am.
That's the difference in our stories.

I'm Andie Dominick, writer, wife, and

mom. I've been diabetic since I was nine years old. My older sister
was diagnosed with diabetes years before I was. I used to think it
was fun to play with her used needles — fun, until the needles were
mine and I had to use them every day, for real. I don't want to be a
famous diabetic writer or a poster child for diabetes. I don't want
to hang out with a lot of diabetic people and I don't want to spend
much time seeing doctors either. I manage my diabetes and my
life just fine. But despite what I want, I still have to see doctors and
nurses.

What This Patient Wants

I want the relationship on my terms.
People don't understand
   that you are paying someone for a service,
   to give advice.
You should control
   how you use that service
   and I guess what advice you take.
That's touchy.
I'm paying them
   and then I get the advice
   and I'm like (laughing), I don't know.
I see it like cut and dry economics.
And then in other ways,
   I want this kind of personal relationship.

Hmm . . .
I'm trying to think of questions doctors ask.
"How have your blood sugars been?" (laughing)
Always that question.
The question I would rather hear
   or would like to hear in addition to that,
   is about non-medical stuff.

It's like they could simply ask,
    "How was your trip here?"
I think that's all I crave, you know, not everything
    revolving around diabetes.

It would seem really easy
    for the doctor to jot
    any simple personal anecdote,
    in my chart and ask about it.
It really connects me with them
and I'm much more able to receive advice
from people I feel are thinking of me
    as a person
                rather than just
                        the next patient.
It is body language.
It is the way someone leans towards you or
    stares at his chart, or
                        makes eye contact.
It's touch.
It's knocking on a door before entering.
Basic respect things.
A perfect example is a physician who talks to you
    before you have your clothes on,
    especially with a woman.
Do you know what I mean?

It's really just a matter of being nice,
    listening, and
    making people feel like
they have some control.

If you want to know what people think,
go sit in a waiting room and
just listen.

I am Sekou Sundiata, a poet, music and

theater artist, and teacher. In 1999, my manager gave me a kidney.
I was the least likely person to need a transplant. I was healthy and
athletic. But in the late 1990s, I was always fatigued. When I finally
saw my internist, he sent me to a nephrologist because my kidney
function wasn't what it should be. The nephrologist gave me a diagnosis — focal glomerulosclerosis, which was frightening, but at least
I had an explanation.

By the next spring, my blood pressure was out of control. I was
having vasospasms, which felt like my gray matter was sneezing or
like a power surge in reverse. I didn't have a center of gravity. The
world seemed to be hard and soft, liquid and solid. Walls just melted
away; the world felt fluid. I was afraid I would be stuck in this spin-
ning liquid reality forever.

Some medications controlled my blood pressure but caused side
effects — edema and dizziness — which immobilized me. Finally, my
doctor hit on using Vasotec and minoxidil and stuff started turning
around, but my kidneys were pretty much shot. I was ready to face
that *if* I had my mind intact, but not if my mind was all spastic and
sneezing.

Over time, I learned that my human narrative and drama — you
know, what was happening to me and what it meant to me — wasn't
written down anywhere in my medical chart. I think my narrative is
as important as what they write in the charts.

Educated Decision

The nephrologist gave me a description of
    hemodialysis and peritoneal dialysis.
I barely grasped it intellectually.
He gave me some pamphlets about PD,
    but I knew something about hemodialysis,
    just in general,
        you know, how you pick up stuff.

I knew that the difference was
     I didn't do hemodialysis myself.
And my whole career as a patient was just that.
     I don't do this myself.
     I come to you.
The most I do is go home and take the pill
     you tell me to take.
I don't hook myself up,
     and drain stuff in,
     and drain stuff out,
     and monitor.
It would be easier for me
     to come in;
               get it done;
                         go home.

The nephrologist's nurse called me and said,
     "Look, you know,
     PD is not for everyone,
     but for some people,
     it's a superior form of dialysis."
She knew the way I lived
     and that I wanted to keep touring and promoting my music.
She kind of tricked me.
She knew if she took me through the hemodialysis unit,
     I would change my mind.
And sure enough, I did.

What's Shakin'?

They put me on the Prograf
     to prepare me for the transplant.
For some reason the tremors
     started in the hospital.
I was in there for three weeks and, oh man,

I thought I'd never get out
   because my creatinine
      was creeping down.
If it was 2.8,
      the next morning it would be
   2.7.
It was just torturous.
It's not like I could do something
   to make it come down.
Finally, the doctor said,
"You can go home."
I started crying.

This one nurse who I really bonded with
   started preparing for me to leave.
She gave me all these medications
   that I didn't know by shape or by color.
There were so many of them.
I was afraid to leave with them in the bag.
I was afraid I would put the wrong med
   in the wrong slot in the weekly pill box.
I tried to put the pills into the slots but
   my hand was shaking.
I couldn't even get them out of the bottles.
I was so frustrated.
She kept coming in — almost like kicking me out —
   saying, "You're not ready yet?"
We had had such a good relationship
   but, for whatever reason, she needed the bed.
It was the first time I had that kind of pressure.
I was like, "Boy, I've been here three weeks,
I've gone through two surgeries, and now
you want to kick me out in an hour."
I felt she handled that really poorly.

Seeing Patients

When my transplant surgeon came in on rounds
and he had residents with him,
he addressed me
   like he knew me,
   like he knew something
     about me,
     about my life.
He conveyed that to them.
"Were you able to do any writing today?"
He'd just take a minute.
I felt he saw me.

Some of the residents who came in without him
   had that attitude.
Not all of them, but a number of them did.
I could see that by modeling that behavior
   they were being trained.
At least they had a model.

Asking Questions

My new nephrologist is a very compassionate guy
   who doesn't hesitate to call me at home.
In New York it's difficult to get to your doctor
   after the office visit.
But my nephrologist calls me back.
He'll call me if something comes up in the labs
   that he wants me to pay attention to,
even if it's not urgent.
Yeah, I'm very fortunate.
He always wants to know
   what I'm teaching,
   what my students are like.

I had heard this term on television —
on one of those medical shows — about percussing your chest.
As a poet who's into music
that was such an interesting term.
So I asked him, "What does it mean
to percuss the chest? What can you tell by doing that?"
"Well, if there's fluid,
it sounds different
than if there's no fluid."
It was really, you know, for a writer,
really wonderful stuff to hear.
I ate this stuff up.

Good Idea

With some doctors
you don't even want to ask questions,
especially if it could seem like you're second-guessing.
Meaning, you've looked something up on the Internet or
you've seen something, and you say,
"Well, what about this instead of that?"
With some doctors that's not even an option.
Both my transplant surgeon
and my nephrologist have been open.
In fact my surgeon changed one of my medications
because of a question I asked.
He said, "That's a good idea;
we should try that."
It was a major medication too.
I've asked him about other medications
and he just said, "No, I don't think that's a good idea."
And he would say why.
But he changed one!

Breaking the Ice

I can remember being in bed
and doctors coming into my room on rounds.
Doctors I didn't even know,
coming to me and not even introducing themselves.
Or in another instance, the doctor saying,
"Good morning," introducing himself,
but not waiting for a response.
He went right on to move the robe and jab me,
not saying anything.

I hate that.
It makes me feel like a specimen.
So I wouldn't feel that way,
I would try, from time to time,
to break the ice by saying,
"Is it cold outside today?"
Or, you know,
anything.

Speaking Their Language

I didn't learn medical language
only to communicate with doctors.
It gave me a sense of power too.
Using medical language with doctors
was kind of like using my high school French
when I went to Paris.
Let me put it this way.
Some doctors would encourage me,
help me along.
I felt they were open to my questions
because when they used words I didn't understand,
I would say, "Well, what's that?"
and they would explain.

Then there were other people
who could tell, of course,
that I didn't know much and they would be like
almost insulted that I would even try.
It was as if they were saying,
"Leave that to me.
Leave that kind of talk to me.
You just had swollen ankles.
You didn't have edema.
Let me talk about edema."

That's the way it was
when I used medical language.

Talking about a Feeling

I'll tell you about someone
    who had the mask on —
turns out I took her personality
    the wrong way.

When I was in the hospital for the transplant,
the kidney stopped working.
I had to have hemo.
The nurse taking care of me
during the treatment
was very matter of fact.
She was unsmiling, you know,
very take charge.
I was like, "Boy, this is a cold fish right here."
Towards the end of the session,
    she came over to disconnect me and said,
"You're going to do fine."
I was startled.
"Really, what makes you say that?"
"I see this often.

Sometimes the kidney just stops working,
and you get dialysis
and it jump-starts the kidney again.
That just happens.
You're going to be fine."
I was like,
   Wow!
   Is this the same person?

She was talking,
   she was talking about a feeling.
She didn't have any science.
She was just letting me in
   on her feeling,
     her sense of it.
That was really nice.
It made such a difference.

Different Narratives

The doctors' narrative in the chart
   is the objective and rational narrative.
That tells you certain things.
Personal narratives can convey
   a sense of what those things mean
   in the life of the patient.
If my creatinine is high,
   I may have to go back in the hospital.
So, that's one level of meaning.
But there's another level of meaning
   that translates into my life.
What do you mean my creatinine is high?
Am I going into rejection?
What does it mean to reject
   if I have a kidney
   from a living, nonrelated donor

and my greatest fear is
    losing the kidney she gave me?
That doesn't just mean
    I'm going back in the hospital.
That's rough.

The personal narrative does that.

I'm Natalie Kusz.
When I was six years old my family moved to Alaska. The first winter there, I turned seven and my dad got a job on the oil fields at Prudhoe Bay. My mom drove into town every day to get water or do laundry. She told me I had to go to the neighbors' house if she wasn't home when I got off the school bus. On January 10, 1970, I came home from school before mom arrived from doing her errands. As I walked to the neighbors' house, their new huskies snarled and hurled themselves at me. I was nearly past the dogs when one of them caught my hair and pulled me down. Mom later found me in the snow. I had more than 100 lacerations on my face and shoulders. My left cheekbone and eye were gone. I was so badly hurt, the doctors told my parents I probably wouldn't live. Mom prayed that I would die. But I lived. I spent a lot of time in the hospital as a kid; I've had more operations than I can count. For a while in college, I was a pre-med student, but later opted to become a writer instead. As an adult, I helped my dad with his health care, and I have had my own health issues as well.

Nostalgia

When I was a kid, I liked the hospital
for the most part.
I was a princess,
a precious jewel.
I got all kinds of attention.
I was comfortable;
nobody made fun of me.
It was everybody's job to look after me.

Even today,
my blood pressure goes down
when I go to a doctor's office
because I'm so glad to be where
it is somebody's job to fix me.

I used to own two hospital johnnies
and I walked around in them all the time.
So, you know,
I sometimes feel very nostalgic.

Fat

I've been diagnosed as fat
                    for so many things.
I've been diagnosed as fat
                    when I had torn ligaments.
I've been diagnosed as fat
                    when I had tendonitis in my wrist.

At first it was "Let's not do surgery
    until you've lost some weight.
Come back when you're 30 pounds thinner,"
    which was hard to hear
    but it didn't sound insurmountable.
Later I started to be afraid to go to the doctor
because I am always accosted about this.

My younger sister, Bethel,
    who basically is my identical twin
    but she has two eyes and is thin,
doesn't have much of a problem with that.
Though for a while, she was fat,
    and then
she could not get taken seriously.

It's Brilliant

The osteopath in my hometown,
I mean, he's in like this hick place
dealing with pretty stoic,
medically mistrusting farm guys half the time
or mechanics or whatever.
I would have expected that I would be
really dismissive of his style
but somehow I'm not.
You get in there
and he says, "What's wrong with you?"
You tell him.
He says, "I'm going to send Claudia or whoever
in to do these three things.
We are going to take some blood;
we're going to do this and this and this.
Then I'll come back and talk to you."
When he comes back,
he has looked at all your stuff.
He sits down.
I mean, this man has no time on his hands
but he still does it.
He goes through the entire history
of everything he has thought
when he was looking at your chart.
He says, "Well, you have this blood count.
So my first thought was
that means she doesn't have this.
But then you said you have this other pain
in this other place
so I looked at this second thing
and that makes me think this."

By the time he tells people the verdict,
the diagnosis,
everybody believes everything he says.

I've never heard of anybody
giving him a hard time about anything.
People who refuse to take medicine
will do whatever he tells them to do.
People who are hypochondriacs
will go home with no medication
when he says, "I think it's just heartburn."

He delineates his process
which makes everything he does palatable.
And because he doesn't tell you up front
what he thinks the end product is, you know,
there is no sense that he's telling you a bunch of stuff
to convince you of what he already had in mind.
It is very effective.
It works for very uninformed patients
and it works for pretty sophisticated ones.
I feel educated myself.
I've been thinking a lot about why it works
and I'm not exactly sure what label to put on it.
But it is brilliant. It is just brilliant.

I am Fitzhugh Mullan, a physician,

educator, activist, administrator, and editor. When I was thirty-two, I took a chest X-ray on myself because I had a chronic cough. I was stunned to find a cauliflower-like density the size of a grapefruit near my heart. During a mediastinoscopy, the surgeon took a bite out of my innominate vein and I needed an emergency thoracotomy. I woke up in the ICU to learn that a seminoma was encasing the vital structures of my chest. After I recovered from the operation I had radiation and chemotherapy. I learned later that my right phrenic nerve was accidentally cut in the chaos of the operation. Nobody told me I was going to have an aftermath like that. And I had even more complications — superior vena cava syndrome — and also sternal osteoradionecrosis, which happens sometimes when bones are irradiated. At that time there were no textbooks for doing a sternectomy and replacing it with a full-thickness skin flap. It was kind of ad lib.

Before all this happened, I knew that sooner or later all doctors become patients. I just didn't think I would cross over so soon.

Taking Responsibility

After my book *Vital Signs* came out,
I sent my surgeon a copy.
He called me immediately
and he was very laudatory.
He thought I got the story right.
He said, "But you don't know
what happened at the biopsy, do you?
You didn't think I did the biopsy.
Well I did.
I did the biopsy;
I've done hundreds of those.
There are two approaches,
one suprasternal,
the other through the sternum.

Through the sternum is a little harder
and you're left with a scar.
I just didn't want to put you through that.
So we went suprasternally,
but the exposure is less good.
It's the last time I ever, ever
did one of those."

He took total responsibility for it.
So I felt good about that.
But I can't get around the fact
that it was an error, it shouldn't have happened,
and it has left me with a compromised life.
I mean, it's not like losing a leg,
it's not like being dead.
But it's certainly eating away at my life
in terms of my abilities, my athleticism;
it's just the constant annoyance and worry.
This was a whoopdee-do medical error.

In It Together

I remember vividly
the surgeon who performed the biopsy
                          that went awry
would make rounds on me every day,
spend time with me, encourage me
    not just medically
                but also personally.
I was in the old naval hospital.
At the time they were building
    a new naval hospital —
        the drills and jackhammers
                were banging away.
He said,
    "I'm going to die in that hole."

When I asked what he meant,
he replied,
   "I'm a naval officer. I'll be retired navy.
   I'll come back here to get my medical care.
   I'll probably die in that hospital."
Which was a little bit of a stretch.
On the other hand, it said to me
that he understood
   he was mortal too.
   He was human;
   he was in this struggle with me.
His biology was going to run its course
just like mine was, although
   mine might have been running a little faster
than one would want.

Being a Great Case

I came in to have a skin graft revised.
There was a delay.
I was on a stretcher,
   bundled up, IV running,
   feeling generally shitty.
The plastic surgeon had a team with him,
   probably students or residents.
He was down the hall talking—
   theoretically out of ear shot,
   actually in ear shot.
He kept referring to me as
     a great case.
I was a rare bird.
They were going to have
   an opportunity to do things
       they didn't normally do.

It reinforced that there are two classes,
  those of us who are healthy,
    in white coats,
      calling the shots,

and the great cases.

It was like living a metaphor —
  the metaphor for insensitivity.

Try to Remember

I'm just amazed
  at how awkward the hospital is.
Big teaching institutions
  have their multiple teams,
    and their multiple instructional requirements.
The patient is sort of bounced
                between competing needs.

As a patient, I so often felt like
  a square peg trying to get into
                a round hole.
My needs as a person,
  as a sick person,
weren't always met by the hospital.

Having been a healthy kid,
  I had to learn that there was
                this land of sickness.
Suddenly I was
  a lieutenant or a captain or a colonel
                in this land of sickness,
but I had never actually been sick.
And then I got sick
  and earned all the credentials one could want
                on the other side.

So I try to make medical care
    as customer friendly as it can be.
From time to time, I say to students,
"Try to remember that we are all patients."

That perspective
    is not hard for me to keep,
but I try to pass it along.
Students are still naïve enough
    or young enough
        or uncalloused enough
that they can hear patients.
If I say to residents,
    who are tired and run from pillar to post,
"Wait a minute.
    Does Mrs. Jones understand
        what you have told her?
Have you really addressed her needs?
Have you thought about what she is feeling?
Have you thought about what happens
        when she goes home?"
they reply, "I don't have time for that."
Which is often true.

I am John Hull, a professor of religious education at the University of Birmingham in the U.K. I was born with a condition characterized by asthma, eczema, and congenital cataracts. When I was young the treatment for cataracts was sticking a needle into them to let out the cloudy stuff. Unfortunately, this eventually caused my retinas to be pulled forward and become detached. I had numerous procedures to reattach my retinas but I finally went completely blind when I was in my forties. More recently, I've had some urologic surgery and even acquired a surgical infection with the methicillin-resistant staph bacteria, which I think most people call MRSA. I've been seen by lots of doctors over the years.

Objective Detachment

Once after a retina repair, I very quickly
noticed the telltale black disc
in my peripheral vision.
I had had this so many times.
That's when I ran into resistance,
really quite stubborn resistance.
I went to the Outpatient Clinic and
I overheard a bit of conversation
between a junior doctor and the surgeon.
"Mr. Hull is here."
"Oh, what's wrong with him?"
"He thinks he's got a detachment."
"Oh, he always thinks he's got a detachment."
Another junior doctor
who examined me very carefully
said, "There's no detachment in that eye."
I said, "I can see it.
There is a detachment.
I'm almost certain."
"Well, you have had detachments

in the past,
you may have them
in the future,
but I can assure you,
you haven't got one now."
I knew he was wrong.
But I had to go.

Every day, I would measure the blind spot
and I could see it approaching the macula.
Of course, I was extremely nervous.
I actually sent a letter by recorded delivery
to the surgeon's home address.
I thought I had no alternative.

I finally saw the surgeon, himself.
He was very brisk and terse.
He examined me and said
"I can't see anything."
He stood up.
I looked him in the eye, and I said,
"Look here, when I look at your mouth,
I can't see your eyes."
That turned him on.
Previously I had been saying
"The upper right-hand quartile
is smoothed off with a semi-circular disc
around which there are flashing lights and
through which is a deep-green, opaque, wobbly jelly.
It's moving slowly across the field of vision,
and I didn't move it."
When I looked him in the eye, and said
"I'm looking at your lips.
I cannot see your eyes,"
then he got it.

He looked and looked for a long, long time,
and then he muttered in a very low voice —
I could hardly hear him —
"There is a detachment.
We must operate.
I will transfer you to another consultant."
I said, "That's not necessary.
Your hands are steady as anybody else's and
your skill is as good as anybody else's.
Thanks for the offer."
He said,
"No, no, you've had enough trouble
with your eyes,
you're not having trouble
with your doctors as well."

It Finally Registered

After I became a registered blind person,
I kept on with three monthly
appointments at the eye hospital
for several years.
Nobody quite had the courage
to discharge me.
Ophthalmologists can't face blindness.
To them blindness means
defeat,
and they don't want that.

One day a new consultant,
a young fellow I'd never met, saw me.
He asked, "Do you have any eye sensation?"
"No, none at all."
"Why do you keep coming in here?"
"I don't know.

Why do you keep sending me appointment cards?"
"Would it be OK
if we don't send those any longer?"
"Sure, that would be fine by me."

That's how it happened.
It was the new fella,
the new staff.
The old staff,
I don't know why
they didn't have the heart.

Under Local

My recent urologic surgery
    was a remarkable experience.
It was three and a half hours
    under local anesthetic.
Of course, there was no pain.
But I could feel everything,
    the pulling,
    the tugging.
Sometimes the doctors seemed to be
    jumping on me.
Down in the stem of my brain,
the ancient part was screaming,
    Get the hell out of here
    these guys are cutting your guts out!
But the rational part of my mind was saying,
    Now look, this is silly.
    These guys are just doing their job, and
    you'll be better.

The anesthetic nurse was wonderful.
She sat by my ear
the whole time and

we talked about our kids,
    our jobs,
        what the weather was like.
She was marvelous.

The surgeons were like three guys
    fixing up a car on a Saturday morning.
One of the surgeons calls out,
    "Can I have a six and a half centimeter one please?"
The nurse brings it to him, and he says,
    "No, no, this is too long.
            Try a shorter one.
    No, no, this is too short.
            Show me the such and such,
            the seven point five.
    Ah, yes, this is the one.
            This does the job, yeah."
And he went on and on and on.

At one stage, a surgeon called out,
    "John this is like cutting through old rope."
There was a lull, and then
one of the men said,
    "Do you think this is it?"
And another one said,
    "Hmm, could be, not sure."
Then the other said,
    "No here it is."

I felt like saying,
"Take your time guys."

I am Tracy Thompson.

On December 18, 1968, when I was thirteen, I was hit by a car. I suffered internal injuries, multiple broken bones, and lacerations. The left side of my scalp was torn from my skull. Most of my injuries healed quickly but I was left with a red, jagged scar over a quarter of my face. Even before the accident, bouts of heart-pounding anxiety woke me at four A.M. I hid these episodes from everyone. After the accident, I was really angry but I just stuffed it. Anxiety and depression, what I call "the beast," surfaced and stalked me as an adult. Finally, I couldn't deny it anymore.

Despair creeps up on me, slowly robbing me of joy and concentration. I can't read, which is excruciating for a writer and journalist. When insomnia and really jumpy anxiety set in, I know something bad is going to happen and I need to take measures. Recently, I called my doctor and said, "I need something for a little while. The insomnia is pervasive." And it was like, bing, this light went on in his head, *I've got a drug addict on the phone*. It has been hard as hell to convince doctors that I know what I am talking about and that I am not looking to abuse drugs and that I am willing to work with them. But it is just really hard.

Raving

My gallbladder surgery
was part of a long-running saga.
There wasn't anything wrong with my gallbladder
when they took it out.
I had a small gallstone that was asymptomatic.
Much, much later they realized
endometriosis was causing periodic intestinal obstruction.
But it took them five years to figure that out.
In the meantime,
I wound up in the hospital six times;

I lost count of the times
I went to the emergency room.

Pain and nausea and vomiting
would just come out of nowhere.
I felt so out of control.
I never knew when I was going to be
doubled over with horrible vomiting and pain,
not knowing what had caused it.

Once I got sick in Penn Station
and puked on the floor of the ladies' room.
I wound up at a hospital in New York.
The emergency room was a horror story.
By the time I got there, I was covered with vomit
and they thought I was a street person.
I kept telling them I worked for the *Washington Post*,
and they must have thought I was raving.
They stuck me over in a corner
and didn't pay any attention to me for hours.
I was vomiting the whole time.
Finally, somebody came in
and pushed an NG tube down my nose.
Instant relief.
They sent me upstairs, put me in a ward
with eight other women,
all of whom spoke Spanish.
The NG tube helped for a little while
and then it got bad again.
I was throwing up all night long.
In the end, this orderly, who looked like
he was going through detox himself, showed up.
He gave me a new blanket
and he held a pail under my head
while I vomited some more.
He was the only person
that paid any attention to me.

The next morning when the doctors made rounds,
I told them I had to call my office.
They said, "Oh, what office is that?"
And I said, "The *Washington Post.*"
They suddenly realized
    I wasn't nuts, that
    I had health insurance.
Within about an hour, I had a private room
and life got very different
    very quickly.

Those ladies in the ward felt so sorry for me.
    I could tell.
But when the doctors figured out
    I had insurance, that
    I was employed,
I waved good-bye and
    the ladies never saw me again.
I wondered what kind of care they got
    all the time.
That was really an eye opener.

The Difference

Ultimately, I hooked up with
this gastroenterologist in Washington
whose claim to fame was that he treated
President Reagan's polyps (laughing).
Anyway, he is a really good doctor
and he finally said to me,
"Tracy, are you sure this isn't related to your periods?"
I thought back and realized that it was.

The other doctors all saw my symptoms
in terms of their specialty.
They saw whether or not my symptoms

fit what they knew how to treat.
The gallbladder specialist
found a bad gallbladder.
To a man with a hammer
everything looks like a nail.

What the gastroenterologist did that was different
was that he really listened to me
and he made me feel like he had time to talk,
like he wasn't checking his watch the whole time.
He didn't have time to just sit there
and shoot the shit
but he knew that I could get to the point
and he was willing to wait while I did.
It was my job to pay attention to my body,
to give him as much information as possible,
to get to the point as soon as I could
and tell him what he needed to know.
It was his job to listen to me.
I felt like we had a partnership.
It shouldn't be that hard
but it seems to be.

Problem Patient

I'm not trying to snow you
    with my knowledge.
I'm not trying to be overbearing.
I just want you to recognize
    I'm an educated lay person,
    I'm not some dimwit.
I want you to deal with me accordingly.
I don't try to pass myself off as somebody
    who has a lot of medical knowledge.
I do know about my illness.
I do know a little bit about drugs and therapies.

All I want to do is talk to you
　　like you understand I have a brain.
It is really, really tough
because the minute I say that —
particularly being a woman,
I don't know how it is for men —
I see myself getting knocked into
　　　　　　　　　　　this pigeonhole of "problem patient."
I don't know how they refer to me
　　but I know I am put into

　　　　　　　　　some category.

Assembly Line

Ob/Gyn's seem to be
　　particularly stressed and their offices are crowded.
I quit one Ob/Gyn because every time
I walked into the waiting room
　　there was never a place to sit down.
They were overbooking and it just was —
I would routinely wait an hour
　　before they would get me in the examining room.
Then I would wait another half hour or 45 minutes.
I told them I couldn't do it.
They looked at me kind of like
　　what's wrong with you?
It was mutual incomprehension.

In Ob/Gyn clinics I feel like I'm
　　in that Charlie Chaplin movie
　　on the assembly line.
You have 0.5 seconds to
　　take your drawers off,
10 seconds to
　　get your feet in the stirrups

and tell the doctor what the deal is.
This is unfortunate because you're dealing with
    really intimate topics.

I thought that I had found a good OB
    and then I had a bad experience with him.
I told him I was trying to get pregnant again
    and he put me on Clomid.
I said, "Okay, I'll give this a try
    but when I was on Clomid before
    it precipitated a really bad depression."
He said, "Okay, all right, fine, we'll keep an eye on things."
After about three months,
    Clomid precipitated this awful depression.
I told him, "I can't do this anymore."
He said, "Really, I've never heard of anybody
    being depressed on Clomid."
He even looked it up in his PDR.
    He said, "Well, yeah, it is listed
    but so are hives and convulsions.
    It's really, really rare."
He made me feel like

                            a total idiot.
I left there almost in tears and
    furious at him.

It is so hard to talk to doctors when
    you go all to pieces
because they are not going to listen
    if you are sobbing while you are saying it.
You are on such an unequal footing.

I doubt I'll go back to him again.

Nut Case

When my mom had a stroke,
    her neurologist was just a jerk.
I mean, he knew his stuff
    in terms of the human brain
    but, in terms of people skills,
                        zip.
It was clear to me,
    after mom started to recover her speech,
    that she was profoundly depressed.
I said to him, "Can we do something about that?"
I made the mistake of saying,
    "I've suffered from depression so I know,
    I know it, I know my mother
    and I know this illness
    and I see it on her face."
The minute I said I'd had trouble with depression,
    it was like, "nut case," and he stopped listening.
His eyes just clicked and he said to me,
    "Well, of course she's depressed,
                        she's had a stroke."
I couldn't think of anything to say.
It was like, "Well, of course he's in pain,
                        he's got cancer."
Well, fine.
                        But what are you going to do about it?

Dating Service

This is going to sound trite.
But I think it is important to be
smart and empathetic
at the same time
so that you don't get so carried away

with the technical aspects of the medical problem
that you forget that there is a person there.
That is the part where it sounds trite.
But, you know, when my mom
was in the hospital with her stroke—
and I'm sorry now that I didn't do this—
at one point I was going to get a picture of her
from when she was healthy
and stick it on the wall above her bed
so they could look at it and say,
"This is the person you are talking to,
not this person with drool coming out of her mouth
who can't even talk,
but this person right here."
Maybe they ought to treat doctors' visits
like dating services
where the patient has a flattering photo
on the front of his files
so they could say,
"Oh, okay, here's who this is.
Not this haggard-looking person
with his butt hanging out."
Maybe they ought to have a photographer
in the waiting room so you could just—
I mean, that's facetious
but you get my point.

Border Crossing

When I had a D&C a couple of years ago
I had to show up to the hospital
really early.
You start with the admitting office.
    You give them your card.
    They strap a bracelet on you.
    You have to sit in the wheelchair
                        in order for them to take you to your room.
I remember remarking to my husband
    that it's like you have this passport
                        and you are journeying to a foreign country.
Yeah, it is like journeying
    from the land of the healthy
                        to the land of the unwell.
It is really this distinct sense
    that you are crossing this boundary
    and that once you cross that boundary
                        people treat you differently,
                        they talk to you differently.
It is striking.
You become, somehow,
                        slightly less adult.

It starts with that stupid wheelchair.
    You are not allowed to walk to your room,
    you have this little identifier on your wrist,
    and those stupid hospital gowns.
It seems like they ought to be able to
    come up with a hospital gown
    that would cover up your butt (laughing).

It is one casual indignity after another.
I imagine disabled people live with this
all day every day.

I am Tom Sleigh, a poet with PNH, or paroxysmal nocturnal hemoglobinuria.

This means I have crises when lots of my red blood cells break open, leaving me severely anemic and at risk of strokes and heart attacks. The trouble started when I was twenty-five. I woke up one morning and my urine was black. It felt like a hatchet had come down and, bang, divided my life in two. The person I was had vanished. In a few years, I'll have been alive as many years with it as without it. Outwardly, I lead an almost completely normal life. I notice the PNH only when I get really sick. Then it takes up every fucking second of my day for up to a month. I don't want to be an invalid; I don't want to be dependent on a medical world, which, when I look at it, doesn't value individual lives, even though it is all about trying to save lives. That is one of the main reasons I really try to keep it together, because I don't want to be dependent on medicine.

Nightmare

My mother arranged
   for me to see a doctor who had PNH.
He wouldn't transfuse me.
His experience with PNH was you don't transfuse.
It was so stupid,
   and useless,
     and pointless
       that I was denied transfusions
               because my doctor
   had been through this experience.

He was a good man and a good doctor,
   but it was frustrating and infuriating
   to deal with him because
he didn't have the detachment to step away
   from his case
and look
         at my case.

Everybody thought he would be
 so compassionate.
But I could not get him to listen.
He refused. He was adamant.
He knew it had to be done his way.

It would be a much smarter idea
                    to have a hematologist who did not have
the same disease I was suffering from.

I talked to him two years ago.
It was amazing, utterly amazing.
He said to me,
 "Every time I have a hemolytic episode,
 I think, man, this is it.
 I'm convinced I'll hemolyze down to 19
 and die."
His guard came down.
It was touching and it delighted me.
But on the other hand,
                    boy, what a nightmare it was
to have him treat me.

The Good, the Bad, and the Clueless

There are a lot of good doctors.
There are some bad doctors.
And then there are doctors
 who don't have a fucking clue
 how to deal with human beings.
It is probably not their fault
 because they are overworked.
The system is brutal.
It is brutal to the patient,
 and it is brutal to the doctor.
I couldn't imagine

getting 87,000 phone calls
the way my hematologist does
and not being half crazy.
But he's not.

I am lucky that I have hematologists
who have followed me for years.
I don't see one of them very much
because he cares for me
only during the hemolytic episodes
and he is so busy.
But when I see him,
he is incredibly focused.
He is not my friend,
but damn, he is a good doctor
and he's very compassionate
within the limits of professional compassion.
I don't think there is any shame in that.
There is nothing wrong
with professional compassion.
I'm sure the compassion
he feels for his family
is very different than what
he feels for his patients.
But it is admirable
and you can see he feels it.
Lots of doctors and nurses don't have that.
They are professionally polite.
But compassion?
I don't see it.

My other hematologist has done
a lot of research on PNH.
She keeps me abreast
of what is going on.
So, I have a rudimentary

working knowledge
of hematology.
She has been an utter dream.
Phenomenal.
I have gotten to know her
    as a person.
She has seen me through
    a number of things.
She knows my story.
She gets it in some deep way.

Special Case

I've had   real specialized treatment
    because I'm   a special case.
Everybody wants to have a crack at me.
You are in this bizarre situation
    when you are   a medical anomaly.
In a way that works to your advantage
    when you are in a hospital
        because everybody wants to do the history
                            on the PNH guy,
    so they can say they saw one.
Frankly, at first, I thought that was weird
but now I am grateful
    because the more attention you get
                        the better it is.

Different Languages

The medical profession
has an unbelievably specialized language.
If a patient comes forward
with impressionistic

(you know what I mean)
descriptions of these experiences
and presents it in a way
that doesn't fit the vocabulary,
it is shrugged at and ignored.
Maybe there is no way to incorporate it
into what doctors can do.
Maybe the patients will keep doing it.
But I don't think doctors
are going to listen to it.
For example, when I say,
"A red blood count of 32 feels a lot different to me
than 26, or 27,"
doctors say, "Yeah, whatever floats your boat."
I can see their eyes glazing over,
I can see them brown out.

Somebody Like Me

I think it would be great
if there was a central medical archive
in which there were long edited patient interviews,
anthologies of patients
talking about their experiences.
So that every medical student,
every medical school across the country,
would make a significant place
for this kind of thing.
If doctors were put in contact
with this kind of material,
if they could hear what it cost people spiritually,
and if they knew firsthand from the sound of a person's voice,
or from what their voice sounds like on a page,
the suffering the people they are treating go through,

they could be made more human by it
and more responsive to the people they are treating.

I have thought about proposing
to the medical school at Dartmouth
that somebody like me
teach a course on this stuff
to doctors.
I would love to do that.
I would certainly be the person to do it,
as opposed to doctors
who talk about their experience
as doctors in relationship to patients and
tell other doctors to treat patients humanely.
That just doesn't compute.

There are plenty of people
in my situation who are articulate
who could actually communicate
with that audience
and make a difference.
Whether there is going to be any room
in medical school for it
is a different question.

My name is Louise DeSalvo.

I write, I teach English at Hunter College in New York, and I do research on Virginia Woolf. I have asthma. I am asthmatic. I am a person with asthma. I get asthmatic attacks — oh, whatever. Let me tell you about my pulmonologist.

Self-Prescribing

My pulmonary doctor
was respectful
of the fact that
I was doing all this alternative stuff.
Like it occurred to me,
I did a lot of reading,
it occurred to me
that I needed to build up
the bellows capacity of my lungs.
So it made sense to me
to do aerobic exercise.
So, I prescribed that for myself.
Because my asthma was emotionally triggered,
it made sense to me that I should meditate.
My pulmonologist said, "Keep doing it if it's working.
Keep doing it."
But no one suggested it
as a component
of good health care
for an asthmatic — a person with asthma,
whatever the hell I am.

A Story to Tell

My pulmonologist is absolutely divine,
an old-world man.
You walk into his office.
He traipses in,
greets you,
looks you straight in the eye.
He sits you down
and he sits over there;
takes out a sheet of paper,
you know,
not a chart,
a sheet of paper.
He says "So tell me,"
and starts listening.
He starts writing
and writing and writing
and writes everything.
And as he's writing and listening
I'm suddenly feeling,
you know,
I have a story to tell
about this illness.

Biographical Notes

Marva Dawn is a scholar and writer who considers herself to be a freelance theologian and educator. She serves the global church with Christians Equipped for Ministry, Vancouver, Washington, and is a teaching fellow in spiritual theology at Regent College in Vancouver, British Columbia. She uses her experiences with health problems and health care to illustrate the arguments she makes in her lectures and books, particularly *I'm Lonely, Lord — How Long? Meditations on the Psalms* and *Powers, Weakness, and the Tabernacling of God*, which won an award from *Christianity Today*.

Louise DeSalvo is a writer, scholar, lecturer, an excellent cook, and an aficionada of great food. She is the Jenny Hunter Endowed Scholar for Creative Writing and Literature at Hunter College. After being diagnosed with asthma, she published *Breathless*, which describes how asthma affected her life and the lives of authors such as Marcel Proust, and *Writing as a Way of Healing: How Telling Our Stories Transforms Our Lives*. Her *Vertigo: A Memoir* won a Gay Talese Award for Best Italian American Book 1993–1997. *Feuds and Forgiveness in an Italian American Family* was named a Book Sense Book of the Year for 2004.

An editorial writer for the *Des Moines Register*, **Andie Dominick's** beats include health care, human services, and social issues. In 2004, she won a Best of Gannet Award in the category of Editorials on the First Amendment. Before joining the *Register*'s editorial board in 2001, she taught creative writing in the English department at Iowa State University. Her essay "Pamphlets," in *The Healing Circle: Authors Writing of Recovery*, describes her early experience with diabetes. Another essay won a Writers' Digest Award, and led to a contract for *Needles: A Memoir of Growing Up with Diabetes*. This won an Alex Award in 1999, given by the American Library Association to honor their selections for the best books for teenagers.

Emily Douglas is the pseudonym of a writer who writes and teaches in the U.S. and abroad. She continues her pursuit of narratives that give voice to the body and good health in every form.

Laura Steele Evans worked for twenty years as a clothing designer for leading skiwear and sportswear companies in the U.S. Before she was diagnosed with breast cancer, she became an amateur mountaineer. After surviving her treatment, she chronicled her experiences with cancer, medical care, and climbing in *The Climb of My Life*, which was a finalist in the 1997 Books for Better Living Award. She was also the first person to climb a major peak after undergoing a bone-marrow transplant, Argentina's 23,000-foot Mount Aconcagua. She founded Expedition Inspiration, which raises money for breast cancer research through walks and climbs. She died of a glioblastoma on October 17, 2000.

Arthur Frank is a professor of sociology at the University of Calgary. After being treated for testicular cancer, he began exploring narratives of illness and the use of narrative in medicine. He has written numerous chapters and scientific articles and given many workshops and invited plenary talks at national and international meetings. Frank chronicles his experience with testicular cancer in *At the Will of the Body: Reflections on Illness* and discusses the role of telling stories of illness in *The Wounded Storyteller: Body, Illness, and Ethics*; he recently published *The Renewal of Generosity: Illness, Medicine, and How to Live*. He serves on several editorial boards and is an elected Fellow of the Hastings Center and of the Royal Society of Canada. Among his numerous honors was being selected to deliver the R. A. Goodling Lectures at Duke University Divinity School.

Michael Gearin-Tosh was an English scholar, teacher, and writer. He was a junior lecturer at Magdalen College, Oxford, from 1964 to 1965, research fellow at Saint Catherine's College, Oxford, from 1965 to 1971, and tutorial fellow in English literature from 1971 to 2005. He excelled as a teacher, and several former students helped him with his health regimen after he became ill. He was also involved in theater and haute couture. His book, *Living Proof: A Medical Mutiny*, described his diagnosis with multiple myeloma and the alternative therapy he chose instead of chemotherapy or a bone-marrow transplant. When diagnosed with myeloma in 1994, he was told he had six months to live. He died on July 29, 2005, outliving the doctors' predictions by eleven years.

John Hull is emeritus professor of religious education at the University of Birmingham. He is also an honorary professor of practical theology in the Queen's Foundation for Ecumenical Theological Education, Birmingham, England, where he teaches and does research. He is the general secretary of the International Seminar for Religious Education and Values, which he founded in 1977. He has published numerous books, including *Touching the Rock* and *On Sight and Insight*, which describe the experience of becoming blind as an adult, and *In the Beginning There Was Darkness: A Blind Person's Conversation with the Bible*.

Natalie Kusz teaches creative writing at Eastern Washington University. She previously taught at Bethel College and was the director of the creative writing program at Harvard University. She has published essays in *O, Harper's, McCall's, Threepenny Review,* the *Utne Reader, Real Simple,* and the *New York Times.* She has won a Whiting Writer's Award, a Pushcart Prize, and a General Electric Younger Writers Award and was awarded fellowships from Radcliffe College's Bunting Institute and the National Endowment for the Arts. In 1990, she published *Road Song*, which recounts her family's move from California to Alaska, their struggle to build a warm home, and their lives after she was mauled by a neighbor's husky. *Road Song* has been translated into German and Chinese and was included in *500 Great Books by Women: A Reader's Guide*.

Steve Kuusisto is the author of *Only Bread, Only Light*, a collection of poems from Copper Canyon Press and of the memoirs *Planet of the Blind* and *Eavesdropping*. He holds a dual appointment at the University of Iowa in English where he teaches courses in creative nonfiction and in the College of Medicine where he serves as a public humanities scholar. He speaks widely on diversity, disability, education, and public policy. His essays and poems have appeared in numerous anthologies and literary magazines including *Harper's*, the *New York Times Magazine*, *Poetry*, and *Partisan Review*. He is currently working on a collection of prose poems for Copper Canyon Press entitled *Mornings with Borges* as well as a collection of political poems about disability.

Nancy Mairs is a poet and an essayist. Many of her essays describe her struggles to maintain her physical and mental health. She is the author of *Plaintext, Ordinary Time: Cycles in Marriage, Faith, and Renewal,* and *Carnal Acts*. In *Waist-High in the World: A Life among the Nondisabled* and *A Troubled Guest: Life and Death Stories*, she takes on the taboo subjects of disability and death. She continues to write and lecture despite her disability. She was awarded a National Endowment for the Arts Fellowship in 1991. She also serves on the boards of ARTability and the Arizona Center for Disability Law.

Richard McCann is the author of *Mother of Sorrows*, an award-winning collection of stories, and of *Ghost Letters*, a collection of poems. His work has appeared in such magazines as the *Atlantic, Esquire, MS*, and *Tin House*, and in numerous anthologies, including *Best American Essays* and *The O. Henry Prize Stories 2007*. For his work, he has received awards and fellowships from the Guggenheim Foundation, the National Endowment for the Arts, the Rockefeller and Fulbright foundations, Yaddo, and the Fine Arts Work Center in Provincetown. He is currently working on a memoir, *The Resurrectionist*, in which he explores his experiences as a liver transplant recipient. He lives in Washington, D.C., where he is a professor at American University.

Christina Middlebrook is a licensed clinical social worker, a practicing Jungian analyst, and a member of the C. G. Jung Institute of San Francisco. She recounts her experience with a bone-marrow transplant for breast cancer in the book *Seeing the Crab: A Memoir of Dying before I Do*, which won the 1997 Books for a Better Life Award for Memoir.

Faye Moskowitz is professor of English and former chair of the English department at George Washington University. She has published *And the Bridge Is Love: Life Stories; Whoever Finds This: I Love You; A Leak in the Heart: Tales from a Woman's Life*; and *Peace in the House: Tales from a Yiddish Kitchen*. She edited *Her Face in the Mirror: Jewish Women on Mothers and Daughters*. Her essay "Because I Could Not Stop for Death," in *The Healing Circle: Authors Writing of Recovery*, describes her mother's death from breast cancer, her own fear of getting cancer, and her diagnosis and treatment for breast cancer. Her work has appeared in many anthologies, journals, magazines, and newspapers in the United States and Israel.

Fitzhugh Mullan is a physician who suffered serious complications from his treatment for cancer. He described his experiences in *Vital Signs: A Young Doctor's Struggle with Cancer* and in "The Seasons of Survival," which was published in the *New England Journal of Medicine*. He also published *White Coat, Clenched Fist: The Political Education of an American Physician; Politics and Plagues: The Story of the United States Public Health Service*; and *Big Doctoring in America: Profiles in Primary Care*. He is a contributing editor to *Health Affairs* where he is the editor of the "Narrative Matters" section. He worked for years in the U.S. Public Health Service. Currently he is the Murdock Head Professor of Medicine and Health Policy at George Washington University, and he practices pediatrics at a clinic in Washington, D.C. He is the cofounder of the National Coalition for Cancer Survivorship.

Teresa Richards is the pseudonym of a writer who wants to move beyond her hip replacements. She has published her work in numerous magazines and anthologies and has won several awards for her writing.

Oliver Sacks is clinical professor of neurology at the Albert Einstein College of Medicine, adjunct professor of neurology at the NYU School of Medicine, and consultant neurologist to the Little Sisters of the Poor. He has published numerous books exploring how people adapt to neurological diseases. *A Leg to Stand On* describes his experience with a disabling neurological condition that complicated his recovery after he tore his quadriceps tendon from his patella. His books have won numerous prizes and have been translated into twenty-two languages. His work has been published in the *New Yorker* and the *New York Times* as well as in medical journals. He has received a Guggenheim Fellowship.

Richard Selzer was a surgeon on the faculty of Yale School of Medicine for many years; he retired at age fifty-eight so he could write full time. *Raising the Dead: A Doctor's Encounter with His Own Mortality* described his intensive treatment for Legionnaire's disease. He has published essays and short stories in *Redbook, Esquire,* and *Harper's,* and is the author of many books. His stories and essays are often used in medical education to trigger discussions about ethics in medicine and have inspired many physicians to write their own stories. He has won a Pushcart Prize, a National Magazine Award, and an American Medical Writers Award.

Tom Sleigh is a poet and playwright. He teaches at Dartmouth College and in the graduate creative writing program at Hunter College. A poem in *Waking* and essays in *Interview with a Ghost* and *The Healing Circle: Authors Writing of Recovery* provide glimpses into his life with paroxysmal nocturnal hemoglobinuria. His poems have appeared in many journals and magazines, including the *New Yorker.* His books of poetry have won many prizes, and he has won an Academy Award from the American Academy of Arts and Sciences, a Shelley Award from the Poetry Society of America, and an Individual Writer's Award from the Lila Wallace Fund. He has also received grants from the Guggenheim and the Ingram Merrill foundations and from the National Endowment for the Arts.

Jane Smiley is a writer and a horsewoman. She taught at Iowa State University in Ames from 1981 to 1996. She has published essays in *Vogue,* the *New Yorker, Harper's,* and the *New York Times Magazine.* Her novels include *The Age of Grief, The Greenlanders, Ordinary Love and Good Will, A Thousand*

Acres, which won the Pulitzer Prize in 1992, *Moo, Horse Heaven, Barn Blind*, and, most recently, *Ten Days in the Hills*. She has written several nonfiction books on subjects as disparate as horse racing, the life of Charles Dickens, and craftspeople in the Catskills. Her essay, "Two Plates, Fifteen Screws," in *The Healing Circle: Authors Writing of Recovery*, describes her broken leg and its effect on her life and health.

Richard Solly is a senior acquisitions editor with Hazelden Publishing. His essay "The World Inside" appears in *The Healing Circle: Authors Writing of Recovery* and chronicles his ordeal after Crohn's disease caused his bowel to rupture. His new book of poems, *From Where the Rivers Come*, is published with Holy Cow! Press. His writing has won numerous fellowships and awards, including the Minnesota State Arts Board Award, the Bush Foundation Artist Fellowship, the Loft-McKnight Award, and the Pearl Hogrefe Fellowship from Iowa State University. He lives in St. Paul, Minnesota.

Sekou Sundiata was a jazz musician, poet, and spoken-word artist. He taught literature at Eugene Lang College, the New School, in New York City. He released several albums, including *longstoryshort* and *The Blue Oneness of Dreams*. His solo performance piece *blessing the boats* relates his experience with uncontrolled high blood pressure, kidney failure, and a kidney transplant. He was a Sundance Institute Screenwriting Fellow, a Columbia University Revson Fellow, and a Master Artist-In-Residence at the Atlantic Center for the Arts. Sundiata was featured in Bill Moyers' PBS series on poetry, "The Language of Life." He died July 18, 2007, of congestive heart failure.

Mary Swander, Distinguished Professor of English at Iowa State University, writes poetry, nonfiction, fiction, plays, and radio essays. Her poems, essays, short stories, and articles have appeared in the *Nation, National Gardening Magazine*, the *New Republic*, the *New Yorker*, the *New York Times Magazine*, and *Poetry*. She has won numerous awards, including a Whiting Award, a National Endowment for the Arts grant for the literary arts, two Ingram Merrill fellowships, the Carl Sandburg Literary Award, and the Nation-Discovery Award. She wrote in detail about her health problems and her interactions with health-care providers in her memoirs *Out of This World: A Journey of Healing*; *The Desert Pilgrim: En Route to Mysticism and Miracles*; and "The Fifth Chair," in *The Healing Circle: Authors Writing of Recovery*.

Tracy Thompson is a journalist who began her career at the *Atlanta Constitution*, where she was a finalist for a Pulitzer Prize for investigative reporting. She later became a staff writer for the *Washington Post*, where she continues to work. After she was hospitalized for depression, she "went public," publishing an essay in the *Post* about her long struggle with the disease. She subsequently shared her experiences and insights with a larger audience in her book-length memoirs *The Beast: A Journey through Depression* and *The Ghost in the House: Motherhood, Raising Children, and Struggling with Depression*.

Bibliography

Benedict. *St. Benedict's Rule for Monasteries*. Translated by Leonard J. Doyle. Collegeville, MN: Liturgical Press, 1948.

Dawn, Marva J. *I'm Lonely, Lord — How Long? Meditations on the Psalms*. Grand Rapids: Wm. B. Eerdmans, 1998.

———. *Powers, Weakness, and the Tabernacling of God*. Grand Rapids: Wm. B. Eerdmans, 2001.

DeSalvo, Louise. *Breathless: An Asthma Journal*. Boston: Beacon Press, 1997.

———. *Writing as a Way of Healing: How Telling Our Stories Transforms Our Lives*. New York: HarperSanFrancisco, 1999.

Dominick, Andie. *Needles: A Memoir of Growing Up with Diabetes*. New York: Scribner, 1998.

Evans, Laura. *The Climb of My Life: A Miraculous Journey from the Edge of Death to the Victory of a Lifetime*. New York: HarperSanFrancisco, 1996.

Foster, Patricia, ed. *Minding the Body: Women Writers on Body and Soul*. New York: Anchor Books, 1995.

Foster, Patricia, and Mary Swander, eds. *The Healing Circle: Authors Writing of Recovery*. New York: Plume, 1998.

Frank, Arthur W. *At the Will of the Body: Reflections on Illness*. New York: Houghton Mifflin, 1991.

———. *The Wounded Storyteller: Body, Illness, and Ethics*. Chicago: University of Chicago Press, 1995.

Gearin-Tosh, Michael. *Living Proof: A Medical Mutiny*. New York: Scribner, 2002.

Hull, John M. *Touching the Rock: An Experience of Blindness*. New York: Pantheon, 1991.

———. *On Sight and Insight: A Journey into the World of Blindness*. Oxford: Oneworld, 1997.

———. *In the Beginning There Was Darkness: A Blind Person's Conversations with the Bible*. London: SCM Press, 2001.

Kusz, Natalie. *Road Song*. New York: Farrar, Straus and Giroux, 1990.

Kuusisto, Stephen. *Planet of the Blind: A Memoir*. New York: Dial Press, 1998.

———. *Only Bread, Only Light: Poems*. Townsend, WA: Copper Canyon Press, 2000.

Mairs, Nancy. *Plaintext*. Tucson: University of Arizona Press, 1986.

———. *Remembering the Bone House: An Erotics of Place and Space*. New York: Harper and Row, 1989.

———. *Ordinary Time: Cycles in Marriage, Faith, and Renewal*. Boston: Beacon Press, 1993.

———. *Waist-High in the World: A Life among the Nondisabled*. Boston: Beacon Press, 1996.

———. *A Troubled Guest: Life and Death Stories*. Boston: Beacon Press, 2001.

McCann, Richard. "The Resurrectionist." *Tin House* 1 (1999): 113–122.

Middlebrook, Christina. *Seeing the Crab: A Memoir of Dying before I Do*. New York: Anchor Books, 1996.

Mullan, Fitzhugh. *Vital Signs: A Young Doctor's Struggle with Cancer*. New York: Farrar, Straus and Giroux, 1982.

Norris, Kathleen. *The Cloister Walk*. New York: Riverhead Books, 1996.

Price, Reynolds. *A Whole New Life: An Illness and a Healing*. New York: Atheneum, 1994.

Rosenbaum, Marcy E., Kristi J. Ferguson, and Loreen A. Herwaldt. "In Their Own Words: Presenting the Patient's Perspective Using Research-based Theatre." *Medical Education* 39 (2005): 622–631.

Sacks, Oliver. *A Leg to Stand On*. New York: Harper and Row, 1987.

Selzer, Richard. *Raising the Dead*. New York: Whittle Books, 1994.

Sleigh, Tom. *Waking*. Chicago: University of Chicago Press, 1990.

———. *Far Side of the Earth: Poems*. New York: Houghton Mifflin, 2003.

———. *Interview with a Ghost*. St. Paul: Graywolf Printing, 2006.

Smith, Anna Deavere. *Fires in the Mirror*. New York: Anchor Books, 1993.

———. *Talk to Me: Listening between the Lines*. New York: Random House, 2000.

Solly, Richard. *From Where the Rivers Come: Poems*. Duluth, MN: Holy Cow! Press, 2006.

Swander, Mary. *Out of This World: A Woman's Life among the Amish*. New York: Viking, 1995.

Thompson, Tracy. *The Beast: A Journey through Depression*. New York: Plume, 1996.

———. *The Ghost in the House: Motherhood, Raising Children, and Struggling with Depression*. New York: HarperCollins, 2006.

Williams, William Carlos. "The Practice." In *The Autobiography of William Carlos Williams*. New York: New Directions, 1951.

Author and Title Index

Subject Index